Gastroenterology

Editors

RICK KELLERMAN
LAURA MAYANS

PRIMARY CARE: CLINICS IN OFFICE PRACTICE

www.primarycare.theclinics.com

Consulting Editor
JOEL J. HEIDELBAUGH

December 2017 • Volume 44 • Number 4

ELSEVIER

1600 John F. Kennedy Boulevard • Suite 1800 • Philadelphia, Pennsylvania, 19103-2899

http://www.theclinics.com

PRIMARY CARE: CLINICS IN OFFICE PRACTICE Volume 44, Number 4
December 2017 ISSN 0095-4543, ISBN-13: 978-0-323-55294-3

Editor: Jessica McCool
Developmental Editor: Colleen Dietzler

Primary Care: Clinics in Office Practice (ISSN: 0095–4543) is published quarterly by Elsevier Inc., 360 Park Avenue South, New York, NY 10010-1710. Months of issue are March, June, September, and December. Periodicals postage paid at New York, NY and additional mailing offices. Subscription prices are $232.00 per year (US individuals), $451.00 (US institutions), $100.00 (US students), $283.00 (Canadian individuals), $511.00 (Canadian institutions), $175.00 (Canadian students), $355.00 (international individuals), $511.00 (international institutions), and $175.00 (international students). Foreign air speed delivery is included in all *Clinics* subscription prices. All prices are subject to change without notice. POSTMASTER: Send address changes to *Primary Care: Clinics in Office Practice*, Elsevier Periodicals Customer Service, 11830 Westline Industrial Drive, St. Louis, MO 63146. Customer Service Health Sciences Division, Subscription Customer Service, 3251 Riverport Lane, Maryland Heights, MO 63043. **Customer Service: 1-800-654-2452 (U.S. and Canada); 314-447-8871 (outside U.S. and Canada). Fax: 314-447-8029. E-mail: journalscustomerservice-usa@elsevier.com (for print support); journalsonlinesupport-usa@elsevier.com (for online support).**

Reprints. For copies of 100 or more, of articles in this publication, please contact the Commercial Reprints Department, Elsevier Inc., 360 Park Avenue South, New York, NY 10010-1710. Tel. 212-633-3874; Fax: 212-633-3820; E-mail: reprints@elsevier.com.

Primary Care: Clinics in Office Practice is covered in *MEDLINE/PubMed (Index Medicus)* and *EMBASE/Excerpta Medica, Current Contents/Clinical Medicine, and ISI/BIOMED.*

Contributors

CONSULTING EDITOR

JOEL J. HEIDELBAUGH, MD, FAAFP, FACG
Clinical Professor, Departments of Family Medicine and Urology, University of Michigan Medical School, Ann Arbor, Michigan

EDITORS

RICK KELLERMAN, MD
Professor and Chair, Department of Family and Community Medicine, KU School of Medicine–Wichita, Wichita, Kansas

LAURA MAYANS, MD, MPH
Assistant Professor, Department of Family and Community Medicine, KU School of Medicine–Wichita, Wichita, Kansas

AUTHORS

EDWARD AGABIN, MD
Assistant Professor, Department of Family Medicine, Medical College of Georgia, Augusta University, Augusta, Georgia

JUSTIN BAILEY, MD, FAAFP
Associate Professor, Department of Family Medicine, UW School of Medicine, Seattle, Washington; Director of Endoscopy, Family Medicine Residency of Idaho, Boise, Idaho

DEE ANN BRAGG, MD
Faculty, Via Christi Family Medicine Residency, Clinical Instructor of Family and Community Medicine, KU School of Medicine–Wichita, Wichita, Kansas

KIMBERLY L. COLLINS, MD
Assistant Professor, Department of Family Medicine, University of Washington, Seattle, Washington

ASHLEY CROWL, PharmD, BCACP
Assistant Professor of Pharmacy Practice, KU School of Pharmacy, Wichita, Kansas

DANIELLE DAVIES, MD
Department of Family Medicine, Teaching Faculty, University of Washington, Seattle, Washington; Faculty, Family Medicine Residency of Idaho, Boise, Idaho

DEAN NATHANIAL DEFREES, MD
Family Medicine, St. Luke's Clinic – Eastern Oregon Medical Associates, Baker City, Oregon

KATHARINE C. DeGEORGE, MD, MS
Assistant Professor, Department of Family Medicine, University of Virginia, Charlottesville, Virginia

DAVID V. EVANS, MD
Associate Professor, Department of Family Medicine, University of Washington, Seattle, Washington

ROBERT FREELOVE, MD
Department of Family and Community Medicine, KU School of Medicine–Wichita, Wichita, Kansas; Smoky Hill Family Medicine Residency, Salina, Kansas

JEANETTA W. FRYE, MD
Assistant Professor, Department of Internal Medicine, Division of Gastroenterology and Hepatology, University of Virginia, Charlottesville, Virginia

GRETCHEN IRWIN, MD, MBA
Associate Professor, Department of Family and Community Medicine, KU School of Medicine–Wichita, Wichita, Kansas

RICK KELLERMAN, MD
Professor and Chair, Department of Family and Community Medicine, KU School of Medicine–Wichita, Wichita, Kansas

TERESA KHOO, MD
Senior Resident Physician, Family Medicine Residency in Palm Springs, University of California, Riverside, Palm Springs, California

THOMAS KINTANAR, MD
Clinical Associate Professor, Indiana University School of Medicine, Lutheran Health Services, Fort Wayne, Indiana

EMILY MANLOVE, MD
Assistant Professor of Family and Community Medicine, KU School of Medicine–Wichita, Wichita, Kansas

LAURA MAYANS, MD, MPH
Assistant Professor, Department of Family and Community Medicine, KU School of Medicine–Wichita, Wichita, Kansas

DANIEL F. McCARTER, MD
Associate Professor, Department of Family Medicine, University of Virginia, Charlottesville, Virginia

STEVEN NGUYEN, MD
Senior Resident Physician, Family Medicine Residency in Palm Springs, University of California, Riverside, Palm Springs, California

LISA K. ROLLINS, PhD
Associate Professor, Department of Family Medicine, University of Virginia, Charlottesville, Virginia

TOMOKO SAIRENJI, MD, MS
Assistant Professor, Department of Family Medicine, University of Washington, Seattle, Washington

AARON SINCLAIR, MD
Assistant Clinical Professor, Department of Community and Family Medicine, University of Kansas School of Medicine, Wichita, Kansas

WILLIAM R. SONNENBERG, MD, FAAPF
Titusville Area Hospital, Titusville, Pennsylvania; Assistant Clinical Professor, Penn State College of Medicine, Hershey, Pennsylvania

KIM M. STEIN, MD
Assistant Professor, Department of Family Medicine, University of Virginia, Charlottesville, Virginia

PATRICK H. SWEET, MD
Family Medicine, Health Sciences Assistant Clinical Professor, University of California, Riverside, Palm Springs, California

ASIF TALUKDER, MD
Surgical Resident, Department of Surgery, Medical College of Georgia, Augusta University, Augusta, Georgia

JENNIFER THUENER, MD
Assistant Professor, Department of Family and Community Medicine, KU School of Medicine–Wichita, Wichita, Kansas

JASON VARGHESE, MD, ThD
Assistant Professor, Department of Family Medicine, Medical College of Georgia, Augusta University, Augusta, Georgia

ANNE WALLING, MB, ChB
Professor, Department of Family and Community Medicine, KU School of Medicine–Wichita, Wichita, Kansas

THAD WILKINS, MD, MBA
Professor, Department of Family Medicine, Medical College of Georgia, Augusta University, Augusta, Georgia

Contents

Gastroesophageal reflux disease (GERD) is a gastrointestinal motility disorder that results from the reflux of stomach contents into the esophagus or oral cavity resulting in symptoms or complications. The typical symptoms of GERD are heartburn and regurgitation of gastric contents into the oropharynx. GERD affects quality of life and may cause erosive esophagitis, esophageal strictures, and Barrett esophagus, a precursor to esophageal adenocarcinoma. GERD is a clinical diagnosis and is most effectively treated with proton-pump inhibitors (PPIs). Long-term use of PPIs is associated with bone fractures, chronic renal disease, acute renal disease, community-acquired pneumonia, and *Clostridium difficile* intestinal infection.

The prevalence of gallstones is 10% to 15% in adults. Individuals with acute cholecystitis present with right upper quadrant pain, fever, and leukocytosis. Management includes supportive care and cholecystectomy. The prevalence of choledocholithiasis is 10% to 20%, and serious complications include cholangitis and gallstone pancreatitis. The goal of management in individuals with choledocholithiasis consists of clearing common bile duct stones. Acute ascending cholangitis is a life-threatening condition involving acute inflammation and infection of the common bile duct. Treatment includes intravenous fluids, analgesia, intravenous antibiotics, and biliary drainage and decompression. Biliary dyskinesia includes motility disorders resulting in biliary colic in the absence of gallstones.

Nonalcoholic fatty liver disease (NAFLD) defines a condition of hepatic steatosis with or without hepatic injury. NAFLD is increasing in prevalence worldwide and presents a public health burden. Most patients are asymptomatic, although some present with fatigue and right upper quadrant pain. NAFLD is discovered incidentally when patients have elevated liver enzymes or fatty liver is seen on imaging modalities. Imaging studies

cause of cancer death before the 1930s to the 13th leading cause of cancer death now. Conversely, esophageal cancer is increasing faster than any other cancer. Screening for esophageal and gastric cancer is not practical in the West, but screening for colon cancer is gratifying for the patient and physician.

The bacteria and fungi in the human gut make up a community of microorganisms that lives in symbiosis with humans, engaging in numerous diverse interactions that influence health. This article outlines the current knowledge on emerging topics in gastroenterology, including microbiome and probiotics, fecal microbiota transplantation, cyclic vomiting syndrome, eosinophilic esophagitis, and microscopic colitis.

PRIMARY CARE:
CLINICS IN OFFICE PRACTICE

THE CLINICS ARE AVAILABLE ONLINE!
Access your subscription at:
www.theclinics.com

Erratum

Errors were made in the September 2017 issue of *Primary Care: Clinics in Office Practice* on pages 413, 414, 417, 421, and 422 in "Managing Polypharmacy in the 15-Minute Office Visit" by Demetra Antimisiaris and Timothy Cutler.

On page 413, "Pharmacy and Medication Management Program" in the affiliation for Demetra Antimisiaris should have been listed as "Polypharmacy and Medication Management Program."

On page 414, "and medication reconciliation" should have been "to medication reconciliation" in the sentence "For example, the Physician Quality Reporting System and the Medicare Access and CHIP Reauthorization Act implemented by the Centers for Medicare and Medicaid Services list several measures that evaluate appropriate medication management as an integral part of outcomes ranging from management of neuropsychiatric symptoms of dementia, plan of care for falls, urinary incontinence plan of care, diabetes control, statin therapy for prevention of cardiovascular disease, and medication reconciliation postdischarge" and "polypharmacy PIMs" should have been "potentially inappropriate medications (PIMs)" in the sentence "The challenges of appropriate management of medications in older adults can be broken down into the following areas: multimorbidity, polypharmacy PIMs in the elderly, underuse of medications, and adherence and access to medications."

On page 417, "PIM" should have been "PIMs" In the sentence "Scan for PIMs for elderly patients by consulting criteria regarding PIM and appropriate medication use in older adults, such as the Beers criteria and START and STOPP criteria."

On page 421, the sentence "The data-gathering aspect can be done as much as possible before the 15-minute office visit with system implementation of medication reconciliation protocol" should have been "The data-gathering aspect can be done as much as possible, before the 15-minute office visit, with systemic implementation of medication reconciliation protocols."

On page 422, "data that from postmarketing surveillance" should have been "data from postmarketing surveillance" in the sentence "Older adults are more susceptible to unexpected adverse outcomes with new-to-market drugs due to lack of physiologic reserve and lack of data that from postmarketing surveillance."

https://doi.org/10.1016/j.pop.2017.09.003
0095-4543/17
primarycare.theclinics.com

Foreword

Bugs, Drugs, and the Unknown

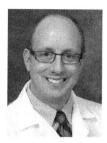

Joel J. Heidelbaugh, MD, FAAFP, FACG
Consulting Editor

One of my students recently asked: "When are they going to develop new drugs for gastrointestinal diseases? How many of these chronic diseases can be cured? Patients suffer, they don't feel well, they take pills, and many don't change their eating habits. It seems quite challenging to improve their quality of life." That same student extolled a vegan lifestyle, as a result of her father being diagnosed with colon cancer at an early age, a sister with celiac disease, and another sister with irritable bowel syndrome. She admitted modest intentional weight loss, more energy, and no reportable gastrointestinal concerns of her own. Seeing many patients with upper and lower, organic, and functional gastrointestinal disorders, it has become a whirlwind of complexity in management and understanding of both cause and effect and prevention.

Treatment of many gastrointestinal diseases has evolved dramatically since I trained 2 decades ago. I remember in the 1990s when new histamine-2 receptor antagonists and proton inhibitors were released and then became available over the counter. Prices plummeted, yet antisecretory medications still remain in the top 3 categories of medications used worldwide. The evidence is strong; they work well, but research has shown us multifactorial causes of gastroesophageal reflux disease and dyspepsia. Hepatitis C, formerly "non-A/non-B hepatitis," exploded in prevalence over the last few decades, especially in people born between 1945 and 1965. Once an indolent disease that was diagnosed late in the course of the disease with little hope for treatment, we now have drugs with very high success rates of complete eradication and tolerable side effects. When I trained, I learned that irritable bowel syndrome was a "diagnosis of exclusion" and was poorly understood, and it meant that everything else had been ruled out. Now, we have clear diagnostic criteria and a panoply of dietary and pharmacotherapeutic options that have proven efficacy.

Gluten: don't eat it, right? Organic foods? *Real* organic foods? Probiotics? Vegetarian? Flexitarian? This diet, that diet: what should we be recommending to our

Prim Care Clin Office Pract 44 (2017) xv–xvi
http://dx.doi.org/10.1016/j.pop.2017.09.002
0095-4543/17/© 2017 Published by Elsevier Inc.

patients? I've learned that treating gastrointestinal diseases is certainly not a "*one size fits all*" model. The future of gastroenterology will continue to uncover a more clear understanding of how we absorb nutrients, which ones we need more and less of, what constitutes our own intestinal microbiome, and how our endocrine systems drive and react to nutrient requirements and depletion. Moreover, the impact of taking multiple medications daily has a profound impact on our overall gastrointestinal health. A deeper understanding of bugs, drugs, hormones, and factors unknown will transform gut health in the future care of our patients with chronic gastrointestinal diseases.

I would like to thank Drs Kellerman and Mayans for their diligent efforts in compiling a very thorough and evidence-based issue of articles on key topics in gastroenterology. Their talented authors conducted solid research to provide our readers with the most current diagnostic and therapeutic recommendations for common gastrointestinal diseases that primary care clinicians manage in daily practice. I always revel in the new information I learn from the expert compilation of our *Primary Care: Clinics in Office Practice* issues; it is my hope that similar value is received by our readership.

Joel J. Heidelbaugh, MD, FAAFP, FACG
Departments of Family Medicine and Urology
University of Michigan Medical School
Ann Arbor, MI 48103, USA

Ypsilanti Health Center
200 Arnet, Suite 200
Ypsilanti, MI 48198, USA

E-mail address:
jheidel@umich.edu

Preface

Gastroenterology

 CrossMark

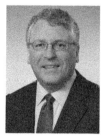 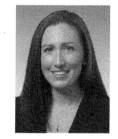

Rick Kellerman, MD   Laura Mayans, MD, MPH
Editors

Primary care physicians frequently see patients with gastrointestinal conditions. Dyspepsia, bloating, nausea, vomiting, constipation, diarrhea, and nonspecific abdominal discomfort are common complaints. Oftentimes digestive disorders are minor conditions that resolve quickly without medical treatment. Others are serious and life threatening; some may be chronic, seriously affecting quality of life. In some situations, minor annoying symptoms may belie a serious underlying problem. When an organic cause for gastrointestinal complaints cannot be identified, the diagnosis is often referred to as "functional."

Over the last decade, dramatic changes have occurred in our understanding of the gastrointestinal system and associated conditions. For example, improvements in the treatment of inflammatory bowel disease and hepatitis C are nothing short of revolutionary. Conditions unrecognized just a few years ago, such as eosinophilic esophagitis and microscopic colitis, have been identified as causes of esophageal food impaction and diarrhea, respectively. Celiac disease, once considered rare, is now commonly considered in the differential diagnosis of abdominal distress. The long-term use of proton pump inhibitors, once considered exceedingly safe, is now recognized to be associated with a variety of significant side effects. The gut bacterial microbiome has been determined to be an important factor in the function of the digestive system and has been implicated in the development of extraintestinal conditions ranging from allergic disease to metabolic disorders and cancer. Fecal microbiota transplantation would have been considered laughable just a few years ago.

Yet, we still have much to learn. Our understanding of the pathogenesis of irritable bowel syndrome (IBS) has improved, but IBS remains a diagnosis of exclusion. We predict that someday in the future, what is now called irritable bowel syndrome will be scientifically explainable, clinically diagnosable, and precisely treatable. Perhaps in the future there will be population-based as well as pharmacologic strategies to stem the developing epidemic of nonalcoholic fatty liver disease associated with

Prim Care Clin Office Pract 44 (2017) xvii–xviii
http://dx.doi.org/10.1016/j.pop.2017.09.001
0095-4543/17/© 2017 Published by Elsevier Inc.

obesity and insulin resistance. The use of probiotics to restore the ideal intestinal microbiome, improve gastrointestinal symptoms, prevent illness, and treat disease will be proven to be fact or fad.

This issue represents a valuable resource for busy primary care physicians on the current status of the epidemiology, pathophysiology, diagnosis, treatment, and management of a variety of gastrointestinal diseases and conditions. We would like to thank the talented authors who dug into the published research and wrote the clinical reviews published in this issue. Each author was dedicated to the project and conscientious in their approach.

We would like to thank Joel J. Heidelbaugh, MD, who asked us to serve as coeditors of this issue. Elsevier staff members Colleen Dietzler, Laura Fisher, Jessica McCool, and Vignesh Viswanathan have been a wonderful and professional team. Thank you all for your assistance in the publication of this issue.

Rick Kellerman, MD
Department of Family and Community Medicine
University of Kansas School of
Medicine-Wichita
1010 North Kansas
3007C
Wichita, KS 67214-3199, USA

Laura Mayans, MD, MPH
Department of Family and Community Medicine
University of Kansas School of
Medicine-Wichita
1010 North Kansas 3001B
Wichita, KS 67214, USA

E-mail addresses:
rkellerm@kumc.edu (R. Kellerman)
lmayans@kumc.edu (L. Mayans)

Gastroesophageal Reflux Disease

Rick Kellerman, MD[a],*, Thomas Kintanar, MD[b,c]

KEYWORDS

- Gastroesophageal reflux disease • Heartburn • Regurgitation • Barrett esophagus
- Upper endoscopy • Proton pump inhibitors

KEY POINTS

- Gastroesophageal reflux disease (GERD) is a gastrointestinal motility disorder that results from the reflux of stomach contents into the esophagus or oral cavity causing symptoms or complications.
- The typical symptoms of GERD are heartburn and regurgitation of gastric contents into the oropharynx.
- Complications of GERD include erosive esophagitis, esophageal strictures, and Barrett esophagus, a precursor to esophageal adenocarcinoma.
- The first-line treatment of GERD is proton pump inhibitors (PPIs).
- Long-term use of PPIs is associated with bone fractures, chronic renal disease, acute renal disease, community acquired pneumonia, and *Clostridium difficile* intestinal infection.

INTRODUCTION

Gastroesophageal reflux disease (GERD) is a gastrointestinal motility disorder that results from the reflux of stomach contents into the esophagus or oral cavity, causing symptoms or complications. The typical symptoms of GERD are heartburn and regurgitation of gastric contents into the oropharynx. Heartburn is the sensation of burning or discomfort behind the sternum. Heartburn may radiate into the neck, is typically worse after meals or when in a reclining position, and may be eased by antacids. Regurgitation is the backflow of gastric contents into the mouth or hypopharynx. Epigastric pain can also be a symptom of GERD. Extraesophageal symptoms of GERD include dental erosions, laryngitis, cough, and asthma.[1,2]

[a] Department of Family and Community Medicine, University of Kansas School of Medicine Wichita, 1010 North Kansas, Wichita, KS 67214, USA; [b] Department of family medicine, Lutheran Health Services, 10020 Dupont Circle Court, Suite 110, Fort Wayne, IN 46825, USA; [c] Department of family medicine, Indiana University School of Medicine, 1110 West Michigan Street, Long Hall Suite 200, Indianapolis, IN 46202, USA
* Corresponding author.
E-mail address: rkellerm@kumc.edu

Prim Care Clin Office Pract 44 (2017) 561–573
http://dx.doi.org/10.1016/j.pop.2017.07.001
0095-4543/17/© 2017 Elsevier Inc. All rights reserved.

EPIDEMIOLOGY

GERD is the most frequent gastrointestinal-related diagnosis made in the United States, and symptoms of gastroesophageal (GE) reflux are the most common indication for upper endoscopic evaluation in the United States.[3] Symptoms of heartburn and regurgitation are more frequently reported by women than by men.[4] The incidence of GERD is 5 per 1000 person-years in the US adult population.[5]

The prevalence of GERD has global variation. The prevalence in North America is 18% to 28% with a sample-size weighted mean of 20%. The prevalence has been increasing in North America, perhaps because of the obesity epidemic.[5]

Some studies may underestimate the prevalence of GERD because of self-treatment with over-the-counter drugs. Other studies may overestimate the prevalence because of variable and imprecise definitions.

GERD has been associated with time off work, a decrease in work productivity, and quality-of-life concerns, such as poor sleep.[6,7]

CLASSIFICATION

The distinction between physiologic reflux of gastric contents into the esophagus and reflux that results in disease (ie, GERD) is a fine line. The physiologic reflux of stomach contents into the esophagus (ie, gastroesophageal reflux, or GER) may be normal in many individuals. Most episodes of GER are brief and do not cause symptoms, esophageal damage, or complications.[1]

The Montreal Definition and Classification Global Consensus Group defines GERD as a condition that develops when the reflux of stomach contents into the esophagus causes troublesome symptoms and/or complications.[1] Symptoms are considered "troublesome" when they adversely affect an individual's well-being. Mild symptoms occurring 2 or more days per week may be considered "troublesome" by some patients.[1]

GERD can be separated into erosive and nonerosive reflux disease (NERD) categories. The erosive category includes symptoms with evidence of esophageal mucosal damage. The NERD category involves symptoms without endoscopic evidence of esophageal mucosal damage. The symptom response rate to proton-pump inhibitors (PPIs) is low in NERD.[1]

The Montreal Consensus Group further delineates GERD into syndromes that are esophageal or extraesophageal based on symptoms and complications.[1]

The esophageal syndromes include subcategories that describe conditions resulting from esophageal injury, including reflux esophagitis, reflux stricture, Barrett esophagus, and esophageal adenocarcinoma. A separate esophageal syndrome category (ie, NERD) includes conditions whereby the patient describes symptoms of regurgitation, heartburn, or chest pain, but there is no evidence of esophageal mucosal injury.[1]

Extraesophageal syndromes associated with GERD include conditions with an established relationship with GERD (eg, dental erosions, laryngitis, cough, and asthma) as well as conditions with a *proposed* relationship with GERD (eg, pharyngitis, sinusitis, idiopathic pulmonary fibrosis, and recurrent otitis media).[1]

RISK FACTORS FOR GASTROESOPHAGEAL REFLUX DISEASE

Many risks factors for GERD have been postulated. The best proven are associations between GERD and body mass index, family history of GERD, and alcohol use.[8]

Other likely risk factors include pregnancy, disordered and delayed esophageal motility from neuropathies and scleroderma, and surgical vagotomy.

Many foods and drugs that decrease lower esophageal sphincter (LES) pressure or cause mucosal irritation have been implicated. Drugs that may be associated with the development of GERD symptoms include drugs such as aspirin and other nonsteroidal anti-inflammatory drugs (NSAIDs), nitroglycerin, calcium channel blockers, anticholinergics, antidepressants, sildenafil, albuterol, and glucagon. Foods that may cause symptoms of GERD include coffee, chocolate, and fatty meals. However, the research on the contribution of these is contradictory. The research is also contradictory regarding the contribution of tobacco smoking to GERD. The evidence for an association with carbonated soft drinks, overeating, and eating rapidly is weak to nonexistent.[9]

PATHOPHYSIOLOGY

The pathophysiology of GERD is multifactorial. Among the mechanisms that predispose to GERD is impaired and transient relaxation of the LES resting tone, delayed gastric emptying, dysfunctional peristalsis, inadequate esophageal acid clearance, reduced salivation, impaired mucosal resistance, and increased intraabdominal pressure. Relaxation of the LES leads to exposure of the esophagus to gastric acid and other stomach contents, such as pepsin, bile, small intestine fluid, and pancreatic secretions, all potentially injurious to the esophageal mucosa.[9] An "acid pocket," an area of unbuffered gastric acid that accumulates after meals in the proximal stomach immediately distal to the GE junction, may serve as a reservoir for acid reflux into the esophagus.[10]

DIAGNOSIS

GERD is primarily a clinical diagnosis. The 2 clinical symptoms that define GERD are heartburn and regurgitation.

A combination of the symptoms of heartburn and regurgitation is enough to make a presumptive diagnosis of GERD.[1] Unless there are alarm symptoms (eg, dysphagia, odynophagia, weight loss, anemia, gastrointestinal bleeding), empiric medical therapy with a PPI can be recommended for symptoms of GERD and may help in clinically confirming the diagnosis.[11] Unfortunately, the sensitivity of the symptoms of heartburn and regurgitation for predicting the presence of erosive esophagitis is only 30% to 76%, and the specificity is only 62% to 96%.[12] Furthermore, response to PPI therapy as a diagnostic tool for GERD has a sensitivity of 78% and specificity of 54%.[13] Nevertheless, upper endoscopy is not required if the symptoms of GERD are typical, alarm symptoms are lacking, and the patient is not at high risk for complications, such as Barrett esophagus.

If initial PPI therapy fails or if the patient has alarm symptoms or is at high risk for complications (eg, age), upper endoscopy is the preferred method of initial evaluation for GERD. Endoscopy has a high specificity for the diagnosis of esophageal findings consistent with GERD.[14] Routine biopsies of the distal esophagus are not required for the diagnosis of GERD.[11] The usefulness of barium swallow radiographs is limited and is not recommended for the evaluation of GERD. Barium swallow radiographs may be indicated for evaluation of dysphagia or the presence of an esophageal stricture or ring.[11,15]

In some cases, ambulatory esophageal reflux monitoring may be recommended. For example, if the diagnosis of GERD remains in question, there are persistent symptoms of reflux despite optimal treatment, or if surgery is being considered, ambulatory reflux monitoring may be indicated. Ambulatory reflux monitoring may help the clinician correlate symptoms with reflux and document abnormal acid exposure in the esophageal lumen. Ambulatory esophageal reflux monitoring aids in the determination of esophageal acid contact time, the number of reflux episodes, and the relationship of reflux to symptoms. Ambulatory reflux monitoring may be performed with a wireless telemetry capsule or with a transnasal catheter.[11,16]

Ambulatory esophageal reflux monitoring techniques include measurement of the esophageal pH and impedance, and manometry. Esophageal pH monitoring is a direct way of measuring acid reflux into the esophagus. An episode of acid reflux is defined as a drop in the esophageal pH to less than 4. Esophageal impedance monitoring measures the change in resistance to an alternating current between 2 electrodes produced by the antegrade or retrograde movement of a liquid or gas bolus inside the esophageal lumen. Impedance monitoring is especially useful when reflux into the esophagus is not acidic. Esophageal manometry is used to measure intraluminal pressure changes in the esophagus. When used in combination, these tests can provide information on the relationship of the functional transport of an air or gas bolus with manometer-detected esophageal contractions and changes in the intraluminal pH. These changes can be correlated with a symptom diary.[16]

If the patient is not on reflux medication, evaluation should be by direct measurement of changes in the esophageal pH or by a combination of impedance and pH monitoring. If the patient is currently on a PPI or H2-receptor blocker, evaluation should be with both impedance and pH monitoring in order to assess nonacid reflux and its relationship to symptoms.[11,16] Esophageal manometry is not recommended for the routine evaluation of GERD, but may be indicated when surgery is being considered for control of GERD. Manometry can be used to rule out achalasia and scleroderma-like esophagus.[11,16]

Because there is no causal relationship between *Helicobacter pylori* and GERD, screening for *H pylori* is not recommended in the evaluation of GERD unless the patient has concomitant peptic ulcer disease.[17]

DIFFERENTIAL DIAGNOSIS

The differential diagnosis of GERD is wide and includes coronary artery disease. Although GERD is the most common cause of heartburn, a clinical caution is that patients with heartburnlike chest pain who have cardiac risk factors should be considered for a diagnostic cardiac evaluation before beginning a gastrointestinal evaluation.[1,11] The differential diagnosis also includes multiple conditions, such as esophageal motility disorders, gastroparesis, esophageal and gastric cancer, peptic ulcer disease, biliary tract disease, achalasia, eosinophilic esophagitis, and distal esophageal spasm. Other considerations include functional dyspepsia, laryngopharyngeal reflux, food allergies, and rumination syndrome. Esophagitis from pills, caustic agents, and infectious causes should be considered. Dysphagia may be associated with GERD and is considered a warning sign for eosinophilic esophagitis, esophageal obstruction, and cancer.[1]

CLINICAL DECISION SUPPORT TOOLS

Clinical decision support tools may facilitate the diagnosis and promote the management of patients with GERD. A symptom scale may be helpful in making the clinical diagnosis of GERD. Structured management based on a GERD symptom score may improve treatment efficacy compared with standard treatment. Use of a GERD treatment algorithm may be more effective than standard treatment of reducing symptoms and improving quality of life in patients with symptoms of GERD. Paper-and-pencil or computerized decision support tools may be available.[18–20]

MEDICAL MANAGEMENT OF GASTROESOPHAGEAL REFLUX DISEASE

Two recent practice guidelines for the management of GERD have been published by Katz and colleagues[11] in the United States and Iwakiri and colleagues[21] in Japan. The guidelines are complementary.

Table 1 compares the 6 PPIs available in the United States and their use for esophageal-related conditions. **Box 1** outlines the recommendations for initial management of GERD.

Approximately 80% of patients will completely respond to an initial management strategy emphasizing the correct use of PPIs.[11] If symptoms resolve after a 4- to 8-week treatment course with a PPI, the medication may be discontinued. **Box 2** outlines a management strategy for patients who are refractory to the initial management strategy outlined in **Box 1**. Maintenance PPI therapy may be indicated in patients whose symptoms are refractory, incompletely resolved, or recurrent, and in patients with erosive esophagitis or Barrett esophagitis. Some patients with noncomplicated GERD may be managed with on-demand or intermittent therapy with a PPI.[11]

Baclofen is a GABA (b) agonist that has been shown to decrease episodes of GE reflux. Its mechanism of action is through reduction of transient relaxation of the LES. For those who are resistant to medical management with PPIs and who have proven GE reflux on ambulatory esophageal reflux monitoring, a trial of baclofen at a dosage of 5 to 20 mg 3 times a day may be considered. The use of baclofen is limited by the side effects of dizziness, somnolence, and constipation. The US Food and Drug Administration has not approved baclofen for the treatment of GERD, and long-term studies of its efficacy are lacking.[11,22]

MANAGEMENT OF EXTRAESOPHAGEAL GASTROESOPHAGEAL REFLUX DISEASE SYNDROMES

Although GERD is associated with dental erosions, laryngitis, chronic cough, and asthma, these conditions are usually caused by multifactorial processes. Clinicians should not assume these conditions are due to GERD alone. Rather, additional evaluation for non-GERD causes should be undertaken in these patients. It is unclear if aspiration of stomach contents causes GERD-related asthma or if a neural mechanism is at work, perhaps a vagally mediated reflex. Upper endoscopy is not typically recommended as a first-line means to establish a diagnosis of GERD-related dental erosions, laryngitis, chronic cough, or asthma. Rather, an empiric trial of a PPI should be considered to treat extraesophageal symptoms in patients who have typical symptoms of GERD. Nonresponders to a PPI trial should be considered for further diagnostic testing. Surgery for GERD is not typically performed to treat extraesophageal symptoms in patients who do not respond to acid suppression with a PPI.[1]

RISKS OF PROTON-PUMP INHIBITOR THERAPY

PPIs are generally well tolerated. The most common side effects of PPIs include headache, diarrhea, and upset stomach. PPIs should be used with caution in patients with hepatic impairment, and dose reductions are recommended.

Evidence of long-term adverse effects of PPI use has been accumulating. Users of PPIs have rates of chronic kidney disease that are 50% higher than nonusers and higher than those who take H2-receptor blockers. Rates of acute kidney disease and acute interstitial nephritis are higher in PPI users than in nonusers. PPI use is associated with a risk of hypomagnesemia. Patients who take PPIs have a 74% higher risk of developing *Clostridium difficile* infection, probably because of the loss of gastric

Table 1
Proton pump inhibitor use for esophageal-related conditions

Proton Pump Inhibitor	Indication/Dosage	Availability	Comments
Dexlansoprazole (Dexilant)	*Healing erosive esophagitis:* 60 mg QD for up to 8 wk *Maintenance for erosive esophagitis:* 30 mg QD for up to 6 mo *Symptoms from nonerosive GERD:* 30 mg QD for 4 wk	30, 60 mg caps No generic No OTC	Due to release mechanism, can be taken without regard to meals Contents of cap can be sprinkled on food[a] and given immediately Dexlansoprazole is the R-isomer of lansoprazole
Esomeprazole (Nexium)	PO: *Healing erosive esophagitis:* 20–40 mg QD for 4–8 wk *Maintenance for erosive esophagitis:* 20 mg QD *Treatment of GERD symptoms:* 20 mg QD for 4 wk IV: *Treatment of GERD symptoms:* 20–40 mg QD for up to 10 d	20, 40 mg caps 2.5, 5, 10, 20, 40 mg suspension 20, 40 mg injectable No generic No OTC	Take at least 1 h before meals Can give suspension and granules from caps through NG tube. Suspension can be given through G tube. Caps can be opened and contents mixed with food[a] For healing of erosive esophagitis or treatment of GERD symptoms, a second course of therapy can be used if necessary Esomeprazole is the S-isomer of omeprazole
Lansoprazole (Prevacid, Prevacid 24HR [OTC])	*Healing erosive esophagitis:* 30 mg QD for up to 8 wk *Treatment of GERD symptoms:* 15 mg QD for up to 8 wk *Treatment of heartburn (OTC):* 15 mg QD for 14 d	15, 30 mg caps 15, 30 mg orally disintegrating tablet Generic available OTC available	Take before eating Granules from caps and orally disintegrating tablet can be given through NG tube Contents of cap can be sprinkled on food[a] and given immediately For healing of erosive esophagitis, a second course of therapy can be used if necessary

Drug	Dosage	Availability	Comments
Omeprazole (*Prilosec, Prilosec OTC*)	*Healing erosive esophagitis:* 20 mg QD for 4–8 wk *Maintenance for erosive esophagitis:* 20 mg QD *Treatment of GERD symptoms:* 20 mg QD for 4–8 wk *Treatment of heartburn (OTC):* 20 mg QD for 14 d	10, 20, 40 mg caps 2.5, 10 mg suspension Generic available OTC and generic OTC available	Take before eating Suspension can be given through NG tube or G tube Contents of cap can be sprinkled on food[a] and given immediately May have more drug interactions than other PPIs Omeprazole is also available in combination with sodium bicarbonate (*Zegerid*)
Pantoprazole (*Protonix*)	PO: *Healing erosive esophagitis:* 40 mg QD for up to 8 wk *Maintenance for erosive esophagitis:* 40 mg QD IV: Treatment of GERD with erosive esophagitis: 40 mg QD for 7–10 d	20, 40 mg tabs 40 mg suspension 40 mg injectable Generic available No OTC	Take suspension 30 min before a meal Suspension can be given through NG tube or G tube An additional course might be needed for healing of erosive esophagitis
Rabeprazole (*Aciphex*)	*Healing erosive esophagitis or ulcerative GERD:* 20 mg QD for 4–8 wk *Maintenance for erosive esophagitis or ulcerative GERD:* 20 mg QD *Treatment of GERD symptoms:* 20 mg QD for 4 wk	20 mg tabs No generic No OTC	A second course of therapy can be used for healing of erosive esophagitis, ulcerative GERD, symptomatic GERD

Abbreviations: caps, capsules; G, gastric; IV, intravenous; NG, nasogastric; OTC, over the counter; PO, orally; QD, every day.

[a] Foods commonly used as a vehicle for administration of medication granules include applesauce, mashed potatoes, pudding, yogurt, cottage cheese, and strained fruits and vegetables. *Data from Prescriber's Letter (www.prescribersletter.com) and product package inserts.*

Box 1
Initial management of gastroesophageal reflux disease

1. For patients who are overweight or have recent weight gain, weight loss is recommended.

2. If the patient has nocturnal symptoms, elevate the head of the bed and avoid meals 2 to 3 hours before bedtime.

3. Avoid foods and drinks that trigger symptoms.

4. Eight-week trial of PPIs for symptom relief. There are no major differences in effectiveness between the different PPIs. PPI therapy should be started at once-a-day dosing, before the first meal of the day. If there is inadequate response to once-a-day dosing, consider increasing the dose, adjusting the timing of the dose, twice-daily dosing, or switching to a different PPI.

5. The general recommendation is to take PPIs 30 to 60 minutes before a meal to maximize the inhibition of proton pumps and control of gastric pH. Some PPIs may be taken with meals.

6. Patients who do not respond to PPI therapy should receive additional evaluation (eg, upper endoscopy).

7. If patients have a return of symptoms after the PPI is discontinued, maintenance therapy with a PPI should be considered. If a PPI is required long term, it should be administered in the lowest dose that is effective, including intermittent use or on-demand use. Explain the long-term risk/benefit ratio of PPI use to the patient.

8. Maintenance PPI therapy should be continued in patients with complications, such as erosive esophagitis and Barrett esophagus.

9. H2-receptor antagonist therapy can be used for maintenance therapy if patients do not have erosive disease and experience heartburn relief.

10. For selected patients with objective evidence of nighttime reflux, bedtime H2-receptor antagonist therapy can be added to daytime PPI therapy, although tachyphylaxis may develop after several weeks of use.

11. Therapy for GERD with prokinetic drugs or baclofen is not recommended without a diagnostic evaluation.

12. PPI use in pregnancy is considered safe.

Adapted from Katz PO, Gerson LB, Vela MF. Guidelines for the diagnosis and management of gastroesophageal reflux disease. Am J Gastroenterol 2013;108:313–4; with permission.

---

acidity and resultant bacterial colonization of the gastrointestinal tract. The risk of community-acquired pneumonia is up to 34% higher in PPI users. PPI use has been associated with an increased risk of bone fractures. There is a 33% increased risk of fracture at any site, a 26% increased risk of hip fracture, and a 58% increased risk of spine fracture. The fracture risk increases after PPI use of less than 1 year. Prudent management strategies include education of patients about the risks of PPIs, discontinuation of empiric PPI use if symptoms are not improving, use of conservative and alternative GERD treatment strategies, and reevaluation of the diagnosis if patients are not improving on a PPI.[23]

SURGICAL MANAGEMENT OF GASTROESOPHAGEAL REFLUX DISEASE

Because of the potential serious complications of PPIs, surgical management of GERD may be considered for some patients. Severe symptoms, esophagitis that is resistant to medical management, and the existence of a large hiatal hernia may be

Box 2
Management of patients with gastroesophageal reflux disease who are refractory to initial management

1. Optimize PPI therapy. Counsel patients to take PPIs as prescribed.

2. Perform upper endoscopy to exclude non-GERD causes.

3. Patients with refractory GERD and a negative endoscopic evaluation should be considered for ambulatory esophageal reflux pH and impedance monitoring.

4. Patients who are refractory to PPI treatment with negative testing for reflux are unlikely to have GERD, and PPI therapy should be discontinued.

5. Patients who are refractory to treatment with objective evidence of ongoing reflux as the cause of symptoms should be considered for additional evaluation (eg, manometry) and antireflux therapies, such as baclofen or surgery.

6. Assess for other causes of symptoms in patients with extraesophageal symptoms of GERD who are refractory to PPI optimization.

Adapted from Katz PO, Gerson LB, Vela MF. Guidelines for the diagnosis and management of gastroesophageal reflux disease. Am J Gastroenterol 2013;108:320–1; with permission.

indications for surgical intervention. Noncompliance with medical management and a desire to discontinue medical management may also be considerations for surgical management.[11]

There are several options for surgical management. For obese patients, bariatric surgery should be considered. Weight loss resulting from successful bariatric surgery may result in improvement of GERD, although symptoms may increase in some because of the restricted size of the stomach after surgery. Roux-en-Y surgery may be more effective than gastric banding.[11]

For many other patients, laparoscopic fundoplication is the operation of choice. Patients with the classic symptoms of heartburn and regurgitation who demonstrate a response to PPIs or who have abnormal ambulatory pH studies have the best surgical response rate to laparoscopic fundoplication.[24]

Factors associated with symptom improvement and resolution following laparoscopic surgery include preoperative symptoms of heartburn, male gender, and younger age. On the other hand, preoperative dysphagia, bloating, and esophageal motility problems are negative predictive factors.[24] Patients should be informed of the short-term mortality and morbidity surgical risks associated with laparoscopic surgery. Postoperative complications of laparoscopic fundoplication include difficulty in belching and vomiting, dysphagia, diarrhea, and gas-bloat syndrome. In many patients, these symptoms may improve with time. Many patients continue to require PPI or antacid therapy after laparoscopic surgery.[24] Open surgical Nissen fundoplication is an alternative to laparoscopic fundoplication, with an attendant increase in surgical risks. Careful patient selection is important when considering surgical therapy. Operator selection is equally important. Preoperative ambulatory pH monitoring and manometry are recommended before surgical intervention.[11]

Creative therapies for the treatment of GERD have been developed. These therapies include tightening the LES with endoscopic suturing, stapling, silicone injection, placement of magnetic titanium beads around the LES, and radiofrequency energy delivery to the LES. Electrical pacing of the LES with an implanted pacemaker has been studied. Unfortunately, these techniques do not yet have proven long-term effectiveness.[11,25]

THE RELATIONSHIP OF GASTROESOPHAGEAL REFLUX DISEASE TO *HELICOBACTER PYLORI*

H pylori may induce gastritis and is recognized as a cause of peptic ulcer disease, but *H pylori* is not a cause of GERD. Patients with typical symptoms of GERD do not need to be tested for *H pylori* unless they also have peptic ulcer disease.[11,17] Gastric infection with *H pylori* may provide protection against Barrett esophagus, although the mechanism of this is unclear.[17]

Interestingly, the location of *H pylori*–induced inflammation in the stomach may have an effect of the symptoms of GERD. Predominance of the *H pylori* organism in the antrum of the stomach results in increased gastric acid secretion, an increased risk of duodenal ulcer, and an increase in symptoms of GERD. Eradication of *H pylori* in these patients is likely to improve the symptoms of GERD. In North America, the most common location of *H pylori* infection is the stomach antrum.[17]

On the other hand, predominance of the organism in the corpus of the stomach leads to gastric atrophy, decreased secretion of stomach acid and, possibly, improvement in the symptoms of GERD. Theoretically, eradication of *H pylori* in patients with corpus-predominant *H pylori* may result in an increase of stomach acid secretion and an increase in symptoms of GERD. This theoretic relationship, as of this time, is unproven.[17]

ESOPHAGEAL COMPLICATIONS OF GASTROESOPHAGEAL REFLUX DISEASE

A major complication of GERD is erosive esophagitis, which is characterized by erosions and ulcers of the esophageal mucosa. Although patients with erosive esophagitis may be asymptomatic, they most often have typical symptoms of GERD. The visual appearance of esophagitis has significant heterogeneity. The Los Angeles Esophagitis Classification System is most often used to grade the degree of esophagitis. The Los Angeles system, which uses an A, B, C, D grading system, is based on the number, length, location, and circumferential severity of breaks in the mucosa.[14,26] PPIs are the standard treatment of erosive esophagitis. Grades C and D are generally described as "severe" and have lower healing rates with PPIs than grades A and B. Follow-up endoscopy to assess for healing is indicated in grades C and D and may be considered for grades A and B.[11]

Esophageal strictures are due to scarring of the esophagus from chronic acid irritation and a disordered healing process. Most strictures due to GERD occur at the squamocolumnar junction.[11] Patients may complain of dysphagia and food impaction. The management of esophageal strictures involves care when swallowing food, and esophageal dilatation may be required. Injection of corticosteroids into the stricture may be considered in recalcitrant cases.[11] Stenting of the stricture may be an option, but stent migration, chest pain, bleeding, and esophageal perforation are problems.[27] Acid suppression with a PPI may be helpful, particularly in preventing stricture recurrence.

Barrett esophagus is a complication of GERD that has malignant potential. Barrett esophagus predisposes to esophageal adenocarcinoma. In Barrett esophagus, metaplastic columnar epithelium replaces the stratified squamous epithelium that normally lines the distal esophagus. Histologically, metaplastic columnar epithelium contains mucus-secreting goblet cells. The metaplastic epithelium develops as a consequence of chronic exposure to gastric acid and other refluxed stomach contents. Other risk factors include age more than 50 years, obesity, smoking, hiatal hernia, male sex, and Caucasian race. For unclear reasons, a diet high in fruits and vegetables, gastric infection with *H pylori*, and the use of NSAIDs may provide protection against Barrett esophagus.[28,29]

Barrett esophagus may display evidence of dysplasia, but not all patients with Barrett esophagus have dysplastic changes. Barrett esophagus progresses to esophageal adenocarcinoma in about 0.25% of patients each year. Progression to esophageal adenocarcinoma is more common in patients with high-grade dysplasia and long segments of affected esophagus.[28,29]

Barrett esophagus may be asymptomatic, although many patients will have typical symptoms of GERD. Patients with Barrett esophagus may have esophageal ulcerations, strictures, and hemorrhage. Esophageal fundoplication, endoscopic mucosal resection, laser ablation, mucosal radiofrequency ablation, cryotherapy, and esophagectomy are procedural management techniques sometimes used for the management of Barrett esophagus. It is controversial whether PPIs or H2-receptor antagonists prevent neoplastic progression in Barrett esophagus, although medical treatment might control the symptoms of GER.[28-30]

There are no current screening recommendations for Barrett esophagus. Routine surveillance of patients who have a diagnosis of Barrett esophagus is indicated. The time interval for surveillance is based on the amount of dysplasia.[28-30] A characteristic surveillance plan is to recommend endoscopy every 3 to 5 years for patients who do not have dysplasia. Unless the dysplasia was eradicated, surveillance should be performed every 6 to 12 months for those with low-grade dysplasia, and every 3 months for those with high-grade dysplasia.[30] The Choosing Wisely campaign recommends that for patients diagnosed with Barrett esophagus who have undergone a second endoscopy confirming the absence of dysplasia on biopsy, follow-up surveillance examinations should not be performed in less than 3 years.[31]

REFERENCES

1. Vakil M, van Zanten SV, Kahrilas P, et al. The Montreal definition and classification of gastroesophgeal reflux disease: a global evidence-based consensus. Am J Gastroenterol 2006;101:1900–20.
2. National Institute for Health and Care Excellence. Gastro-oesophageal reflux disease and dyspepsia in adults: investigation and management. Clinical guideline published September 3, 2014. Available at: nice.org.uk/guidance/cg184. Accessed August 20, 2017.
3. Peery AF, Dellon ES, Lund J, et al. Burden of gastrointestinal disease in the United States: 2012 update. Gastroenterology 2012;143(5):1179–87.
4. Kim YS, Kim N, Kim GH, et al. Sex and gender differences in gastroesophageal reflux disease. J Neurogastroenterol Motil 2016;22(4):575–88.
5. El-Serag HB, Sweet S, Winchester CC, et al. Update on the epidemiology of gastro-oesophageal reflux disease: a systematic review. Gut 2014;63(6):871–80.
6. Becher A, El-Serag H. Systematic review: the association between symptomatic response to proton pump inhibitors and health-related quality of life in patients with gastro-oesophageal reflux disease. Aliment Pharmacol Ther 2011;34:618–27.
7. Gerson LB, Fass R. A systematic review of the definitions, prevalence, and response to treatment of nocturnal gastroesophageal reflux disease. Clin Gastroenterol Hepatol 2009;7:372–8.
8. Mohammed I, Nightingale P, Trudgill NJ, et al. Risk factors for gastro-oesophageal reflux disease symptoms: a community study. Aliment Pharmacol Ther 2005;21(7):821–7.

9. Kahrilas PJ. GERD pathogenesis, pathophysiology, and clinical manifestations. Cleve Clin J Med 2003;70(5):S4–19.
10. Kahrilas PJ, McColl K, Fox M, et al. The acid pocket: a target for treatment in reflux disease? Am J Gastroenterol 2013;108:1058–64.
11. Katz PO, Gerson LB, Vela MF. Guidelines for the diagnosis and management of gastroesophageal reflux disease. Am J Gastroenterol 2013;108:308–28.
12. Moayyedi P, Talley NJ, Fennerty MB, et al. Can the clinical history distinguish between organic and functional dyspepsia? JAMA 2006;295:1566–76.
13. Numans ME, Lau J, de Wit NJ, et al. Short-term treatment with proton pump inhibitors as a test for gastroesophageal reflux disease: a meta-analysis of diagnostic test characteristics. Ann Intern Med 2004;140:518–27.
14. Lundell LR, Dent J, Bennett JR, et al. Endoscopic assessment of oesophagitis: clinical and functional correlates and further validation of the Los Angeles classification. Gut 1999;45:172–80.
15. Johnston BT, Troshinsky MB, Castell JA, et al. Comparison of barium radiology with esophageal pH monitoring in the diagnosis of gastroesophageal reflux disease. Am J Gastroenterol 1996;91:1181–5.
16. Hirano I, Richter JE, Practice Parameters Committee of the American College of Gastroenterology. ACG practice guidelines: esophageal reflux testing. Am J Gastroenterol 2007;102:668–85.
17. Chey WD, Leontiadis GI, Howden CW, et al. ACG clinical guideline: treatment of Helicobacter pylori infection. Am J Gastroenterol 2017;112:212–38.
18. Horowitz N, Moshkowitz M, Leshno M, et al. Clinical trial: evaluation of a clinical decision-support model for upper abdominal complaints in primary-care practice. Aliment Pharmacol Ther 2007;26(9):1277–83.
19. Jonasson C, Mourn B, Bang C, et al. Randomised clinical trial: a comparison between a GERD Q-based algorithm and an endoscopy-based approach for the diagnosis and initial treatment of GERD. Aliment Pharmacol Ther 2012;35(11):1290–300.
20. Manterola C, Muñoz S, Grande L, et al. Initial validation of a questionnaire for detecting gastroesophageal reflux disease in epidemiological settings. J Clin Epidemiol 2002;55(10):1041–5.
21. Iwakiri K, Kinoshita Y, Habu Y, et al. Evidence-based clinical practice guidelines for gastroesophageal reflux disease 2015. J Gastroenterol 2016;51:751–67.
22. Koek GH, Sifrim D, Lerut T, et al. Oesophagus: effect of the GABAB agonist baclofen in patients with symptoms and duodeno-gastro-oesophageal reflux refractory to proton pump inhibitors. Gut 2003;52:1397–402.
23. Schoenfeld AJ, Grady D. Adverse effects associated with proton pump inhibitors. JAMA Int Med 2016;176(2):173–4.
24. Oelschlager BK, Quiroga E, Parra JD, et al. Long-term outcomes after laparoscopic antireflux surgery. Am J Gastroenterol 2008;103:280–7.
25. Ganz RA. A review of new surgical and endoscopic therapies for gastroesophageal reflux disease. Gastroenterol Hepatol 2016;12(7):424–31.
26. Armstrong D, Bennett JR, Blum AL, et al. The endoscopic assessment of esophagitis: a progress report on observer agreement. Gastroenterology 1996;111:85–92.
27. Hindy PA. Comprehensive review of esophageal stents. Gastroenterol Hepatol 2012;8(8):526–34.
28. Spechler SJ, Souza RF. Barrett's esophagus. N Engl J Med 2014;371:836–45.
29. Spechler SJ, Fitzgerald RC, Prasad GA, et al. American Gastroenterological Association medical position statement on the management of Barrett's esophagus. Gastroenterology 2011;140(3):1084–91.

30. Shaheen NJ, Weinberg DS, Denberg TD, et al. Upper endoscopy for gastroesto-phageal reflux disease: best practice advice from the clinical guidelines commit-tee of the American College of Physicians. Ann Intern Med 2012;157(11):808–16.
31. Choosing Wisely. American Gastroenterological Association. Five Things Physi-cians and Patients Should Question. Available at: http://www.choosingwisely.org/societies/american-gastroenterological-association/. Accessed April 4, 2012.

Gallbladder Dysfunction: Cholecystitis, Choledocholithiasis, Cholangitis, and Biliary Dyskinesia

CrossMark

Thad Wilkins, MD, MBA[a],*, Edward Agabin, MD[b],
Jason Varghese, MD, ThD[c], Asif Talukder, MD[d]

KEYWORDS

- Acute cholecystitis • Ascending cholangitis • Biliary dyskinesia
- Choledocholithiasis • Cholelithiasis • Functional gallbladder disorder
- Sphincter of Oddi disorders

KEY POINTS

- Individuals with acute cholecystitis present with right upper quadrant pain, fever, and leukocytosis.
- Ultrasound is the test of choice for acute cholecystitis. Management includes supportive care and cholecystectomy.
- Evidence-based guidelines identify the likelihood that a patient may have choledocholithiasis on the basis of these clinical, laboratory, and ultrasound results.
- Acute ascending cholangitis is a life-threatening condition involving acute inflammation and infection of the common bile duct.
- Biliary dyskinesia includes motility disorders resulting in biliary colic in the absence of gallstones. HIDA scan should be performed to assess the ejection fraction of the gallbladder.

INTRODUCTION

Gallbladder disease (GBD) refers to symptoms or complications secondary to the presence of stones in the gallbladder (cholelithiasis) or the common bile duct (CBD) (choledocholithiasis) (**Fig. 1**). According to National Health and Nutrition Examination

Disclosure Statement: The authors have nothing to disclose.
[a] Department of Family Medicine, Medical College of Georgia, Augusta University, 1120 15th Street, HB 4032, Augusta, GA 30912, USA; [b] Department of Family Medicine, Medical College of Georgia, Augusta University, 1120 15th Street, HB 3021, Augusta, GA 30912, USA; [c] Department of Family Medicine, Medical College of Georgia, Augusta University, 1120 15th Street, HB 3010, Augusta, GA 30912, USA; [d] Department of Surgery, Medical College of Georgia, Augusta University, 1120 15th Street, BI 4070 Augusta, GA 30912, USA
* Corresponding author.
E-mail address: jwilkins@augusta.edu

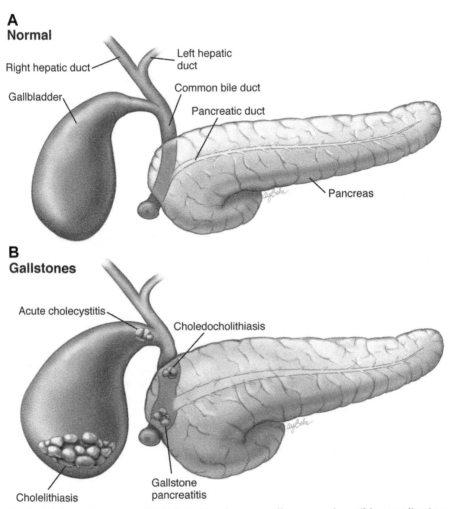

A
Normal

Right hepatic duct

Left hepatic duct

Gallbladder

Common bile duct

Pancreatic duct

Pancreas

B
Gallstones

Acute cholecystitis

Choledocholithiasis

Cholelithiasis

Gallstone pancreatitis

Fig. 1. (*A*) Normal anatomy. (*B*) Gallbladder showing gallstones and possible complications.

Survey III, nearly 20 million adults in the United States have GBD, which is more common in women than men and Mexican-American women have the highest prevalence (26.7%)[1] (**Table 1**). GBD has a low mortality rate (per 100,000) of 0.33 compared with peptic ulcer disease (3.47) and diverticular disease (2.50).[2] The total cost of GBD in the United States is estimated to be $6.2 billion.[3]

GALLSTONES

The prevalence of gallstones is 10% to 15% in adults and is one of the most common and expensive gastrointestinal disorders to treat[4] (**Fig. 2**). Cholesterol gallstones are the most common type in Western societies, accounting for 80% to 90% of stones found at cholecystectomy.[5] Major risk factors for cholesterol gallstones include advancing age, gender, race, family history, pregnancy, and parity.[6] Additional risk factors include high-calorie and low-fiber diets, low physical activity, rapid weight

Table 1
Age-standardized prevalence of gallbladder disease

	Men (%)	Women (%)
Non-Hispanic whites	8.6	16.6
Mexican American	8.9	26.7
Non-Hispanic blacks	5.3	13.9

Data from Everhart JE, Khare M, Hill M, et al. Prevalence and ethnic differences in gallbladder disease in the United States. Gastroenterology 1999;117(3):632–9.

loss, oral contraceptives, metabolic syndrome, and obesity.[6] Nearly 80% of gallstones remain asymptomatic with the risk of pain or complications of 1% to 4% per year.[7,8]

CHOLECYSTITIS
Background

Cholecystitis may be acute or chronic. Individuals with acute cholecystitis (AC) typically present with right upper quadrant (RUQ) pain, fever, and leukocytosis (**Box 1**). There are four forms of AC: (1) acalculous, (2) xanthogranulomatous, (3)

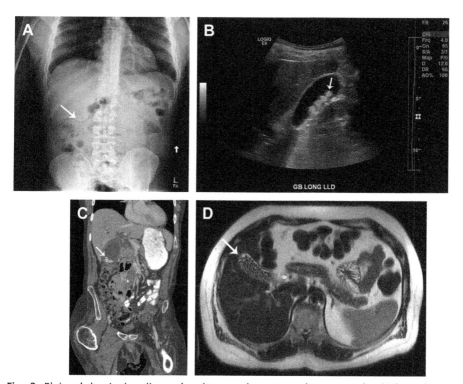

Fig. 2. Plain abdominal radiograph, ultrasound, computed tomography (CT), and MRI showing gallstones. (*A*) Plain abdominal radiograph showing multiple gallstones (*arrow*). (*B*) Transabdominal ultrasound showing four gallstones (*arrow* indicates most caudad stone). (*C*) CT scan showing multiple gallstones (*arrow*). (*D*) MRI shows numerous gallstones (*arrow*).

Box 1
Diagnostic criteria for acute cholecystitis

Clinical manifestations

1. Local symptoms and signs
   a. Murphy sign
   b. Pain or tenderness in RUQ
   c. Mass in RUQ

2. Systemic signs
   a. Fever
   b. Leukocytosis
   c. Elevated C-reactive protein level

3. Imaging findings; confirmation on ultrasound or scintigraphy

Diagnosis

The presence of one local symptom or sign, one systemic sign, and a confirmatory finding on imaging

Data from Strasberg SM. Clinical practice. Acute calculous cholecystitis. N Engl J Med 2008;358(26):2804–11.

---

emphysematous, and (4) torsion of the gallbladder.[9,10] Acalculous cholecystitis is not associated with gallstones and is typically seen in critically ill individuals.[9] Xanthogranulomatous cholecystitis is characterized by thickening of the gallbladder wall and elevated intragallbladder pressure caused by obstructed stones.[9] Emphysematous cholecystitis is characterized by air within the gallbladder wall caused by gas-forming anaerobes.[9] Torsion of the gallbladder results in compromise of the vascular supply, seen most frequently in the elderly, and may result in life-threatening consequences if not promptly treated with cholecystectomy. Chronic cholecystitis occurs after recurrent episodes of AC.

Pathophysiology

AC typically starts with persistent obstruction by a stone resulting in increasing pressure inside the gallbladder causing distention, ischemia, bacterial invasion, and inflammation.[9] Repeated episodes of AC may lead to chronic cholecystitis characterized by thickened gallbladder walls with inflammatory cell infiltration associated with mucosal atrophy and fibrosis.[9]

Diagnosis

There is no single clinical or laboratory finding with sufficient accuracy to establish the diagnosis of AC[11] (**Table 2**). RUQ pain, fever, and vomiting are the most accurate symptoms for AC.[12] Murphy sign and RUQ tenderness are the most accurate examination findings for AC.[12] The initial laboratory work-up includes complete blood count (CBC), liver function tests (LFTs), basic metabolic panel, C-reactive protein level, and blood cultures. The most accurate laboratory abnormalities include elevated total bilirubin, aspartate aminotransferase, alanine transferase, and alkaline phosphatase and leukocytosis.[11]

Imaging

Imaging is necessary to establish the diagnosis of AC and to exclude alternative diagnoses[13] (**Box 2**). The initial imaging modality is abdominal ultrasound because it has

Table 2
Summary of test characteristics for clinical and laboratory findings for acute cholecystitis

Finding	Sensitivity (%)	Specificity (%)	Positive LR	Negative LR
History				
Anorexia	65	50	1.3[a]	0.7[a]
Emesis	71	53	1.5	0.6
Fever (>35°C)	35	80	1.5	0.9
Nausea	77	36	1.2[a]	0.6[a]
RUQ pain	81	67	1.5	0.7
Physical examination findings				
Guarding	45	70	1.5[a]	0.8[a]
Murphy sign	65	87	2.8	0.5
Rebound	30	68	1.0	1.0
Rigidity	11	87	0.9[a]	1.0[a]
RUQ mass	21	80	0.8	1.0
RUQ tenderness	77	54	1.6	0.4
Laboratory				
Alkaline phosphatase >120 U/L	45	52	0.8	1.1
Elevated AST or ALT	38	62	1.0	1.0
Total bilirubin >2 mg/dL	45	63	1.3	0.9
Total bilirubin, AST, and alkaline phosphatase elevated	34	80	1.6	0.8
Leukocytosis	63	57	1.5	0.6
Leukocytosis and fever	24	85	1.6	0.9

Abbreviations: ALT, alanine transferase; AST, aspartate aminotransferase; LR, likelihood ratio.
[a] Calculated by the authors.
Data from Trowbridge RL, Rutkowski NK, Shojania KG. Does this patient have acute cholecystitis? JAMA 2003;289(1):80–6.

good diagnostic accuracy (sensitivity 81%, specificity 83%, positive likelihood ratio [+LR] 4.8, negative LR [-LR] 0.2), is widely available, has shorter examination times, and lacks ionizing radiation[13,14] (**Fig. 3**, **Table 3**). Cholescintigraphy using 99mTc-hepatic iminodiacetic acid (HIDA) is the most accurate test to rule in and to rule out AC (sensitivity 96%, specificity 90%, +LR 9.6, -LR 0.04)[13,14] (**Fig. 4**). Although cholescintigraphy carries no risk of ionizing radiation and provides information limited to the hepatobiliary tract, the contrast is radioactive.[14] Computed tomography (CT) scan and MRI may be helpful in patients presenting with confusing or complicated presentations or when obesity or gaseous distention limits use of ultrasound[13] (**Figs. 5** and **6**). MRI is the preferred test in pregnant patients in whom ultrasound is inconclusive.

Treatment

The management of AC includes supportive care, gallbladder decompression, and gallbladder removal[15] (**Fig. 7**). Supportive care includes intravenous (IV) fluids, nothing by mouth status, and analgesia.[15] Nonsteroidal anti-inflammatory drugs are first-line therapy and are effective for pain secondary to AC.[16,17] Opiate medications are acceptable alternatives for analgesia if nonsteroidal anti-inflammatory drugs are ineffective.[15,18] IV antibiotics are commonly used because 50% to 66% patients with AC

Box 2
Differential diagnosis for gallbladder disease

Acute ascending cholangitis

Acute cholecystitis

Acute hepatitis

Acute pancreatitis

Appendicitis

Cardiac ischemia

Chronic cholecystitis

Fitz-Hugh–Curtis syndrome

Functional gallbladder disorder

Irritable bowel disease

Nonulcer dyspepsia

Peptic ulcer disease

Perforated viscus

Right-sided pneumonia

Sphincter of Oddi dysfunction

Subhepatic or intra-abdominal abscess

---

develop secondary infections.[15] Ursodeoxycholic acid is not beneficial in patients with symptomatic cholelithiasis awaiting cholecystectomy.[19] Low-risk patients may undergo cholecystectomy during the same admission once the inflammation and acute symptoms have improved.[15] A large retrospective study of 95,523 adults who underwent laparoscopic cholecystectomy (LC) within 10 days of presentation with AC found that mortality, postoperative infections, and costs were lower for those who underwent surgery during Days 2 to 5 versus Days 6 to 10.[20] The optimal timing for LC and determination of surgical risks depends on the severity of AC[21] (**Table 4**).

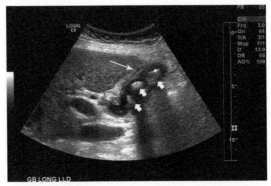

Fig. 3. Ultrasound in a patient with acute cholecystitis. Transabdominal ultrasound from a patient with acute cholecystitis. Ultrasound findings include pericholecystic fluid (*long arrow*) and three large stones (*short arrows*).

Table 3
Summary of diagnostic characteristics for common imaging tests ordered for acute cholecystitis

Imaging Test	Sensitivity (%)	Specificity (%)	Positive LR[a]	Negative LR[a]
Ultrasound	81	83	4.8	0.2
Cholescintigraphy	96	90	9.6	0.04
CT scan[b]	94	59	2.3	0.1
MRI	85	81	4.5	0.2

Abbreviations: CT, computed tomography; LR, likelihood ratio.
[a] Calculated by the authors.
[b] Limited data.
Data from Yarmish GM, Smith MP, Rosen MP, et al. ACR appropriateness criteria right upper quadrant pain. J Am Coll Radiology 2014;11(3):316–22; and Kiewiet JJ, Leeuwenburgh MM, Bipat S, et al. A systematic review and meta-analysis of diagnostic performance of imaging in acute cholecystitis. Radiology 2012;264(3):708–20.

A Cochrane review of six randomized controlled trials including 488 participants with AC and randomized to early LC versus delayed LC found no differences between the groups in terms of mortality, bile duct injury, other serious complications, or the rates of conversion to open cholecystectomy.[22] A Cochrane review of 38 randomized

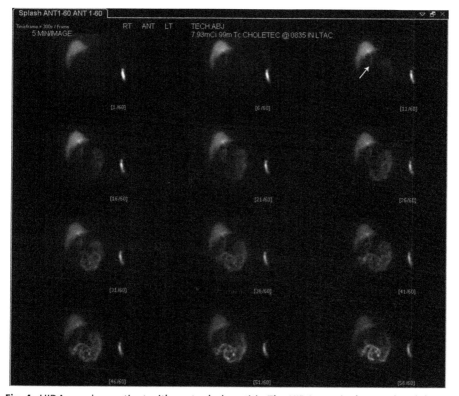

Fig. 4. HIDA scan in a patient with acute cholecystitis. The HIDA scan is abnormal and shows absence of filling of the gallbladder, indicating obstruction of the cystic duct. The duodenum starts to fill with radioisotope at about 15 minutes (*arrow*) and the gallbladder never fills during the course of the 60-minute examination.

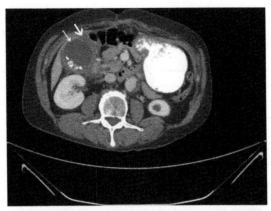

Fig. 5. CT scan in a patient with acute cholecystitis. The CT scan shows a thick-walled and distended gallbladder (*long thin arrow*) with pericholecystic induration (*long thick arrow*). Several gallstones are visualized (*short thick arrow*).

controlled trials including 2338 participants with symptomatic cholelithiasis and randomized to LC versus open cholecystectomy found no significant differences in mortality, complications, and operative time.[23] However, this review found significantly shorter length of stays and convalescence with LC compared with open cholecystectomy.[23]

Percutaneous cholecystostomy may be indicated for patients at high surgical risk with moderate to severe symptoms of AC who are not improving with supportive care (within 72 hours).[24] In critically ill patients, percutaneous cholecystostomy may be superior to LC in terms of decreased length of stay and costs.[24] Emergent surgery is warranted in patients with gangrene, emphysematous cholecystitis, necrosis, perforation, abscess, or worsening clinical status despite supportive therapy.[15]

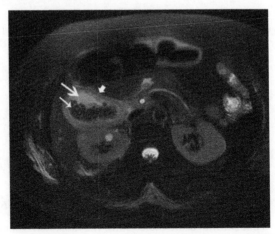

Fig. 6. MRI in a patient with acute cholecystitis. Contrast-enhanced MRI shows numerous gallstones (*long thin arrow*), pericholecystic fluid (*long thick arrow*), and a hyperemic gallbladder wall (*short thick arrow*).

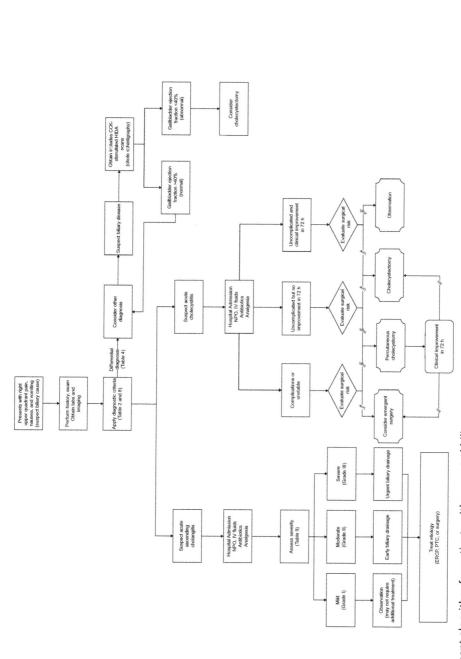

Fig. 7. Treatment algorithm for patients with suspected biliary cause to symptoms. ERCP, endoscopic retrograde cholangiopancreatography; IV, intravenous; PTC, percutaneous transhepatic cholangiography. (*Data from* Miura F, Takada T, Kawarada Y, et al. Flowcharts for the diagnosis and treatment of acute cholangitis and cholecystitis: Tokyo guidelines. J Hepatobiliary Pancreat Surg 2007;14(1):27–34.)

| Table 4 |
| Severity grading for acute cholecystitis |

Grade	Criteria	Comment
Mild (grade 1)	Mild gallbladder inflammation without organ dysfunction	Laparoscopic cholecystectomy may be performed as safe and low-risk procedure
Moderate (grade 2)	Presence of one or more of the following: 1. Elevated white blood cell count 2. Palpable tender mass in the right upper abdominal quadrant 3. Duration of complaints >72 h 4. Marked local inflammation	Likely to be associated with increased operative difficulty to perform a cholecystectomy
Severe (grade 3)	Presence of one or more of the following: 1. Cardiovascular dysfunction 2. Neurologic dysfunction 3. Respiratory dysfunction 4. Renal dysfunction 5. Hepatic dysfunction 6. Hematologic dysfunction	Associated with organ dysfunction; high-risk for surgical complications

Data from Hirota M, Takada T, Kawarada Y, et al. Diagnostic criteria and severity assessment of acute cholecystitis: Tokyo guidelines. J Hepatobiliary Pancreat Surg 2007;14(1):78–82.

CHOLEDOCHOLITHIASIS
Background

The prevalence of choledocholithiasis is 10% to 20% in those with cholelithiasis, although the natural history of CBD stones is not well understood.[25] Serious complications of choledocholithiasis include acute ascending cholangitis (ACC) and gallstone pancreatitis, which are associated with increased morbidity and mortality.[25] CBD stones are the main cause for nonmalignant biliary obstructions.[26] It is estimated that up to 10% of patients who undergo LC may have a CBD stone.[26]

Pathophysiology

Stones found in the CBD may be primary, secondary, residual, or recurrent. Primary stones usually form in the bile ducts in the setting of biliary stasis or physiologic biliary duct dilation, which results in a higher propensity for intraductal stones to form.[26] Most commonly, secondary stones composed of cholesterol form in the gallbladder and pass into the CBD.[26] Residual stones refer to those stones in the CBD that are missed at the time of cholecystectomy but present within 2 years of surgical resection.[25] Recurrent stones develop in the biliary ducts and occur greater than 2 years following surgical resection.[25]

Causes

Major risk factors are related to the development or presence of biliary stasis or infection.[26] Choledocholithiasis is more common in older adults in whom there is physiologic dilation of the CBD. For example, in patients with prior cholecystectomy, the CBD may physiologically dilate up to 10 mm, leading to biliary stasis and the formation of primary stones.[27] Patients with periampullary diverticula are at greater risk for choledocholithiasis.[26] Recurrent infections of the biliary system by organisms, such as *Clonorchis sinensis* or *Opisthorchis viverrini*, cause episodic intraductal inflammation and biliary obstruction.[28] Repeat cycles of obstruction, infection, and inflammation lead to dilation of the extrahepatic biliary ducts, creating the conditions for stasis.

Clinical Presentation

Most patients with uncomplicated choledocholithiasis present with a classic pattern of postprandial epigastric or RUQ pain associated with nausea and vomiting.[29] Pain is not relieved by change in body position and is not related to food intake.[29] The severity of symptoms may depend on the number of stones in the CBD and the size of the stones.[29] Jaundice is caused when a CBD stone becomes impacted in the bile duct.[29] Typically, the pain from choledocholithiasis only resolves if the stone passes spontaneously or is removed endoscopically or surgically.

Diagnosis

In addition to a history and physical examination, the initial evaluation of patients with suspected choledocholithiasis should include LFTs, lipase, CBC, and ultrasound. Evidence-based guidelines identify the likelihood that a patient may have choledocholithiasis on the basis of these results[30] (**Fig. 8**). A recent Cochrane review demonstrated that serum bilirubin elevations twice the upper limit of normal had good diagnostic accuracy for choledocholithiasis (sensitivity 84%, specificity 91%, +LR 9.3, -LR 0.18), whereas elevation of serum alkaline phosphatase twice the upper limit of normal had moderate diagnostic accuracy for choledocholithiasis (sensitivity 92%, specificity 79%, +LR 4.4, -LR 0.1).[31,32] Patients with symptomatic cholelithiasis with a low probability of choledocholithiasis should undergo cholecystectomy alone. Patients with intermediate or high probability of choledocholithiasis benefit from further imaging to further evaluate the need for stone clearance before surgery.

Imaging

Transabdominal ultrasound
A meta-analysis of five studies and 523 participants found good diagnostic accuracy for abdominal ultrasound for CBD stones (sensitivity 73%, specificity 91%, +LR 8.1, -LR 0.3)[31] (**Fig. 9, Table 5**). However, ultrasound more accurately detects dilatation of the CBD based on a small study involving 100 patients undergoing cholecystectomy (sensitivity 96%, specificity 95%, +LR 19.2, -LR 0.04).[33] The probability of a stone in the CBD increases with increasing diameter of the CBD, with a cutoff of greater than 6 mm.[34]

Computerized tomography
Noncontrasted CT has low sensitivity and specificity for choledocholithiasis. There are no meta-analyses on the diagnostic characteristics of CT for choledocholithiasis. The largest study of contrasted CT included 256 individuals with suspected choledocholithiasis and found moderate diagnostic accuracy (sensitivity 77.3%, specificity 72.8%, +LR 2.8, -LR 0.31)[35] (**Fig. 10**). Expense and radiation exposure have limited the use of CT as a first-line diagnostic test for choledocholithiasis.[34]

Magnetic resonance cholangiopancreatography
Magnetic resonance cholangiopancreatography (MRCP) is noninvasive, is rapidly performed, and does not expose patients to ionizing radiation or contrast[3] (**Figs. 11** and **12**). A Cochrane review of 18 studies including 2366 participants demonstrated excellent diagnostic accuracy for the detection of CBD stones by MRCP (sensitivity 93%, specificity 96%, +LR 23.3, -LR 0.07).[41]

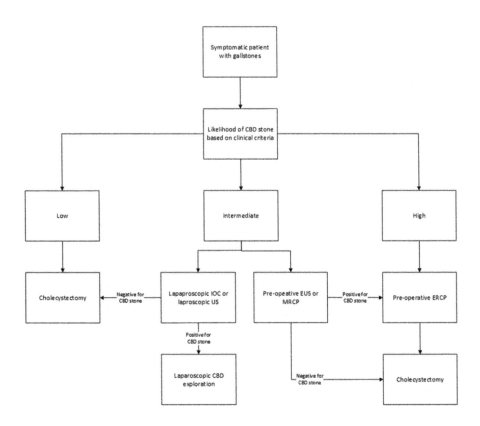

Fig. 8. Diagnostic algorithm for patients suspected of choledocholithiasis. (*Adapted from* Ansaloni L, Pisano M, Coccolini F, et al. 2016 WSES guidelines on acute calculous cholecystitis. World J Emerg Surg 2016;11:25; with permission.)

Endoscopic ultrasound

A Cochrane review of individuals with suspected choledocholithiasis reported that endoscopic ultrasound (EUS) has excellent diagnostic accuracy for CBD stones (sensitivity 95%, specificity 97%, +LR 31.7, -LR 0.05).[41] Results of EUS are operator-dependent, and the procedure may not be widely available in all settings. Complications associated with EUS are rare (0.1%–0.3%). There was no statistical difference between MRCP and EUS.[41] Because MRCP and EUS have high diagnostic

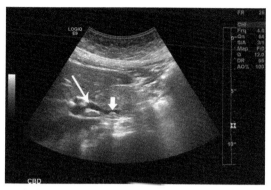

Fig. 9. Transabdominal ultrasound showing dilated common bile duct and stone within common bile duct. A transabdominal ultrasound shows a dilated CBD (*long arrow*) with a stone within the CBD (*short arrow*).

accuracy, individuals with a positive EUS or MRCP should undergo either endoscopic retrograde cholangiopancreatography (ERCP) or surgery with laparoscopic CBD exploration (LCBDE) and those with a negative MRCP or EUS do not need additional testing.[41]

Endoscopic retrograde cholangiopancreatography

ERCP is used to remove CBD stones after sphincterotomy and is the most widely used method for imaging and treating CBD stones (**Fig. 13**). Usually before injecting contrast for imaging, the bile duct is decompressed to decrease the risk of inducing bacteremia with contrast injection. Larger stones (>2 cm) usually require lithotripsy before removal. The success rate with ERCP to clear CBD stones is 90% to 95%.[34] However, ERCP is invasive, requires technical expertise, and includes risks for serious

Table 5
Summary of diagnostic characteristics for common imaging tests ordered for suspected choledocholithiasis

Test	Sensitivity (%)	Specificity (%)	+ LR	− LR	References
Transabdominal ultrasound	73	91	8.1	0.3	Gurusamy et al,[31] 2015
Computerized tomography with contrast	77.3	72.8	2.8	0.3	Tseng et al,[35] 2008
Magnetic resonance cholangiopancreatography	93	94	15.5	0.07	Kaltenthaler et al,[36] 2004
Endoscopic ultrasound	94	95	18.8	0.06	Tse et al,[37] 2008
Endoscopic retrograde cholangiopancreatography	83	99	83	0.17	Gurusamy et al,[38] 2015
Intraoperative cholangiography	99	99	99	0.01	Gurusamy et al,[38] 2015
Laparoscopic ultrasound	95	100	∞	0.05	Machi et al,[39] 2007
Percutaneous transhepatic cholangiography	95	95	19	0.05	Ahmed et al,[40] 2015

Abbreviation: LR, likelihood ratio.

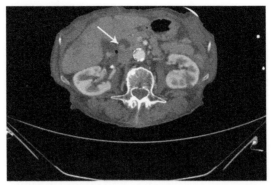

Fig. 10. CT scan showing a distal bile duct stone (*arrow*).

complications, such as iatrogenic pancreatitis (1.3%–6.7%), bleeding (0.3%–2.0%), and perforation (0.1%–1.1%).[34] A Cochrane review of five studies including 318 participants found that ERCP has excellent diagnostic accuracy for choledocholithiasis (sensitivity 83%, specificity 99%, +LR 83, -LR 0.17).[38] Another Cochrane review showed that prophylactic antibiotics before elective ERCP reduced the incidence of bacteremia (number needed to treat = 11) and cholangitis (number needed to treat = 38).[42] There are an increasing number of patients with complex foregut anatomy for whom ERCP cannot be performed, such as those who have undergone Roux-en-Y gastric bypass or Billroth II antrectomy.

Intraoperative cholangiography
Intraoperative cholangiography is performed by insertion of a small flexible catheter into a cystic duct or via the gallbladder and injection of iodinated contrast dye with interpretation by the surgeon at the time of cholecystectomy.[34] Although intraoperative cholangiography may not be technically possible in all cases, is not performed

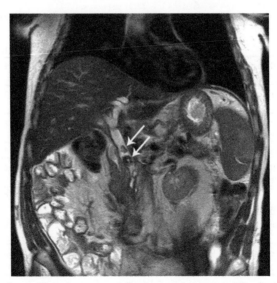

Fig. 11. MRI showing a dilated common bile duct and common bile duct stones (*arrows*).

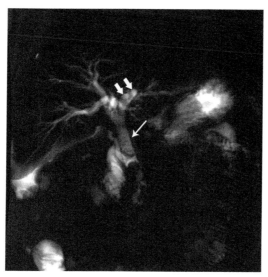

Fig. 12. MRCP showing a dilated common bile duct (*long arrow*) and common bile duct stones (*short arrows*).

by all surgeons, and increases operative time, it has excellent diagnostic accuracy for choledocholithiasis (sensitivity 99%, specificity 99%, +LR 99, -LR 0.01).[38]

Laparoscopic ultrasound

Laparoscopic ultrasound may be performed by the surgeon before LC by passing a flexible ultrasound probe through a standard 10-mm trocar and advancing the probe

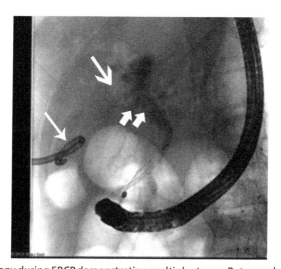

Fig. 13. Fluoroscopy during ERCP demonstrating multiple stones. Retrograde endoscopic cannulization of the anterior and extrahepatic bile ducts injection of contrast material demonstrating multiple stones (*short thick arrows*). Contrast material is seen to retrograde fill via the cystic duct into a decompressed gallbladder filled with stones (*long thick arrow*). The gallbladder is decompressed by the percutaneous cholecystostomy tube (*long thin arrow*).

to the porta hepatis to identify and follow the CBD throughout its course to the duodenum. However, laparoscopic ultrasound may increase operative time and is not widely used by all surgeons.[34] In a small study involving 200 patients, laparoscopic ultrasound had excellent diagnostic accuracy for choledocholithiasis (sensitivity 95%, specific 100%, +LR ∞, -LR 0.05).[39]

Percutaneous transhepatic cholangiography

In patients in whom ERCP is unsuccessful or who have surgically altered anatomy, percutaneous transhepatic cholangiography (PTC) may be used. PTC is performed by an interventional radiologist and may not be available in all clinical settings. A recent review of PTC reported an 8% incidence of complications.[40,43] PTC has excellent diagnostic accuracy for choledocholithiasis (sensitivity 95%, specificity 95%, +LR 19, -LR 0.05).[40]

Treatment

The goal of management in individuals with choledocholithiasis consists of clearing the CBD of stones by either endoscopy or surgery.[25] Treatment options include ERCP with LC or LCBDE with LC. ERCP with LC requires a two-stage approach during a single hospitalization. A recent meta-analysis of 14 studies including 1600 participants concluded there was no difference between the two approaches in terms of successful CBD stone clearance, mortality, morbidity, length of hospital stay, and retained stone.[44] However, only 20% of surgeons in the United States perform LCBDE; therefore, the therapeutic option is often determined by technical expertise and availability.[45]

CHOLANGITIS
Background

ACC is a life-threatening condition involving acute inflammation and infection of the CBD caused by bacteria that ascends from the sphincter of Oddi (SOD) causing Charcot triad of fever, jaundice, and abdominal pain.[46] However, the diagnostic accuracy of Charcot triad for ACC is poor (specificity 95.9%, sensitivity 26.4%, +LR 1.3, -LR 0.16).[9,47] In the most severe form, caused by bacteremia and sepsis, individuals with ACC may have hypotension and altered mental status, a constellation called Reynolds pentad. The male to female ratio for ACC is about equal but ACC is more common in the elderly population and fair-skinned individuals.[46]

Pathophysiology

ACC is usually caused by either increased bacteria or elevated intraductal pressure in the bile duct that allows transfer of bacteria and/or endotoxins into the vascular and lymphatic system. The most common bacteria seen in ACC include: *Escherichia coli* (31%–40%), *Klebsiella* (9%–20%), *Enterococcus* (3%–34%), *Streptococcus* (2%–10%), *Enterobacter* (5%–9%), and *Pseudomonas aeruginosa* (0.5%–19%).[48] There are various etiologies including choledocholithiasis (60%), malignant biliary stricture (9%), iatrogenic biliary stricture (9%), benign biliary stricture (8%), primary sclerosis cholangitis (6%), metastatic liver disease (3%), and primary liver disease (1%).[49]

Diagnosis

In patients in whom ACC is considered, the physician should order a CBC, C-reactive protein, LFTs, basic metabolic panel, international normalized ratio, and blood cultures to help establish the diagnosis and assess the severity. The diagnostic criteria for ACC is based on the Tokyo Guidelines, which has moderate diagnostic accuracy for ACC (sensitivity 91.8%, specificity 77.7%, +LR 4.1, -LR 0.1)[47] (**Box 3**).

Ultrasound and CT scan with contrast help to identify the underlying cause and to exclude other diagnoses. Other imaging modalities include MRCP, MRI, EUS, ERCP, and PTC.[50] Predictive factors for a poor prognosis in ACC include white blood cells greater than 20,000 cells/mm[3], total bilirubin greater than 10 mg/dL, temperature greater than 39°C, serum albumin less than 3.0 g/dL, and age greater than 75.[46,47,51]

Treatment

The severity of ACC ranges from mild to severe[52] (**Table 6**). Treatment options include IV fluids, analgesia, IV antibiotics, and biliary drainage and decompression, depending on the severity.[49] Initially, patients should be given a broad-spectrum antibiotic, then the antibiotic regimen should be tailored to the bacteria found on the blood cultures. In individuals with mild ACC, a first- or second-generation cephalosporin, ampicillin/sulbactam, or piperacillin/tazobactam should be considered.[53] In individuals with moderate to severe ACC, a third- or fourth-generation cephalosporin, ampicillin/sulbactam, or piperacillin/tazobactam should be considered.[53] In individuals with mild ACC, medical treatment may be sufficient, and biliary drainage and decompression may not be required.[54] Patients with ACC who do not respond to medical therapy have moderate disease and require biliary drainage and decompression by ERCP, PTC, or surgery.[54] Patients with ACC and organ failure have severe disease and require organ support, typically in the intensive care unit with urgent biliary drainage performed once the patient has stabilized.[54] ERCP is a safe and effective therapeutic option for patients with ACC during pregnancy.[55]

BILIARY DYSKINESIA
Background

Functional gallbladder disorder (FGD) and SOD are motility disorders of the gallbladder and biliary tract that result in biliary colic in the absence of gallstones.[56] Patients typically present with sharp and crampy pain in the RUQ 30 minutes after a meal.[57] However, patients may be asymptomatic or present with recurrent bouts of nausea, vomiting, cramping, bloating, reflux, or diarrhea.[57] The incidence of these disorders have increased from 5% to 25%, resulting in an increase in the number of cholecystectomies performed.[58] The prevalence of FGD and SOD is unknown; however, SOD is present in up to 1.5% of patients with unexplained biliary pain after cholecystectomy.[59]

Pathophysiology

Biliary dyskinesia occurs when (1) the gallbladder cannot contract properly to secrete bile because of gallbladder dyskinesia or hypokinesia, (2) there is a lack of

---

Box 3
Tokyo Guidelines for acute ascending cholangitis

For suspected acute ascending cholangitis you need two or more of the following:

A. History of biliary disease, fever, chills, jaundice, and right upper quadrant pain

B. Evidence of inflammatory response, abnormal LFTs

C. Biliary dilatation, or evidence of an etiology (eg, obstruction) seen on imaging

Adapted from Kiriyama S, Takada T, Strasberg SM, et al. New diagnostic criteria and severity assessment of acute cholangitis in revised Tokyo Guidelines. J Hepatobiliary Pancreat Sci 2012;19(5):582; with permission.

Table 6
Severity grading of acute cholangitis and treatment

Grade	Grade I	Grade II	Grade III
Description	Mild	Moderate	Severe
Criteria	Responds to initial medical therapy	2 out of 5 predictive factors present	Associated with organ failure
Treatment options	IV antibiotics and biliary drainage/ decompression may not be necessary	IV antibiotics + early biliary drainage/ decompression	IV antibiotics + urgent biliary drainage/ decompression

Adapted from Kiriyama S, Takada T, Strasberg SM, et al. TG13 guidelines for diagnosis and severity grading of acute cholangitis (with videos). J Hepatobiliary Pancreat Sci 2013;20(1):32; with permission.

coordination between gallbladder contraction and SOD relaxation, or (3) the bile cannot flow through the CBD because of a structural or functional outlet obstruction.[56] There is an association between biliary dyskinesia and obesity, which produces a chronic proinflammatory state, fatty infiltration of the gallbladder, and poor motility.[60]

Table 7
Rome IV criteria for the diagnosis of functional gallbladder disorder and functional biliary sphincter of Oddi disorder

Rome IV Criteria for the Diagnosis of Biliary Pain	Rome IV Criteria for the Diagnosis of Functional Gallbladder Disorder	Rome IV Criteria for the Diagnosis of Functional Biliary Sphincter of Oddi Disorder
Pain located in the epigastrium and/or RUQ and all of the following: 1. Builds up to a steady level and lasting 30 min or longer 2. Occurs at different intervals (not daily) 3. Severe enough to interrupt daily activities or lead to an emergency department visit 4. Not significantly (<20%) related to bowel movements 5. Not significantly (<20%) relieved by postural change or acid suppression	1. Must meet criteria for biliary pain 2. Absence of gallstones or other structural pathology	1. Must meet criteria for biliary pain 2. Elevated liver enzymes or dilated bile duct, but not both 3. Absence of bile duct stones or other structural abnormalities
Supportive criteria • Nausea and vomiting • Pain that radiates to the back and/or right infrasubscapular region • Pain that wakes patient from sleep	Supportive criteria • Low ejection fraction on gallbladder scintigraphy • Normal liver enzymes, conjugated bilirubin, and lipase	Supportive criteria • Normal lipase • Abnormal sphincter of Oddi manometry • Abnormal HIDA scan

Data from Cotton PB, Elta GH, Carter CR, et al. Gallbladder and sphincter of Oddi disorders. Gastroenterology 2016. [Epub ahead of print].

Diagnosis

FGD and SOD are diagnoses of exclusion. The initial work-up involves LFTs, lipase, and conjugated bilirubin tests and ultrasound to rule out structural causes (eg, gallstones or tumor). Testing is normal in patients with these disorders. The Rome IV diagnostic criteria should be considered for those suspected to have motility disorders[61] (**Table 7**). Further investigation for FGD includes HIDA scans to estimate gallbladder ejection fraction (EF). Individuals with an EF of less than 40% are considered abnormal, and they are more likely to respond to cholecystectomy[62] (**Fig. 14**). SOD manometry is the gold standard for assessing SOD; however, this invasive procedure is rarely done because of lack of availability and the risk of complications. Other noninvasive tests may be used to diagnose SOD including ultrasonographic measurement of CBD diameter, HIDA scan, and MRCP.[63]

Treatment

Symptomatic treatment of abdominal pain is the cornerstone of nonsurgical therapy. Even though there have been studies showing that opiates produce SOD contraction, IV opiates are still the drug of choice with inpatient treatment. Muscle relaxers and calcium channel blockers are ineffective.[64] Alternative treatments, such as artichokes, celandine, dandelion, and St. John's Wort, may be effective, and typically work through either a cholagogue effect, which promotes the discharge of bile from the biliary system, or a choleretic effect, which increases the volume of secretion of bile

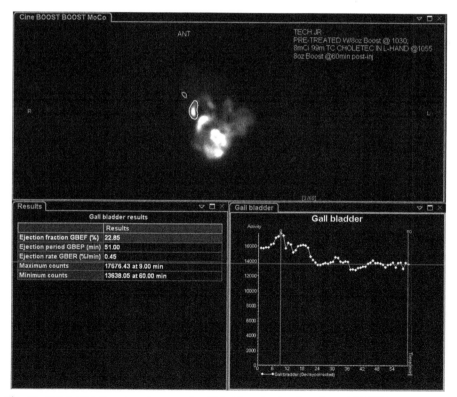

Fig. 14. HIDA scan showing decreased gallbladder ejection fraction of 22.85%.

from the liver.[65] Smoking cessation, eating more frequent meals, avoidance of foods high in fat, weight loss, increased physical activity, and lying on the right side after meals have also been shown to be effective for biliary dyskinesia.[66]

Traditionally, LC as treatment of biliary colic was only viewed effective for those with a low EF on HIDA scan.[67] However, recent studies suggest that LC has relieved biliary colic in patients with both high and low EF, suggesting that EF is only one of several factors when deciding if a patient would benefit from LC.[68] Those who meet the Rome diagnostic criteria with classic biliary symptoms have a high likelihood of successful postoperative outcome, with symptomatic resolution in up to 90% of patients.[69] Individuals with SOD identified through manometry are most effectively treated with endoscopic biliary sphincterotomy resulting in long-term relief in up to 80% of patients.[65]

SUMMARY

GBD is a common problem that often brings patients into the primary care office or the emergency department. AC, choledocholithiasis, ACC, and biliary dyskinesia are the four most common causes of GBD. These disorders are diagnosed by history, physical examination, laboratory tests, and imaging. With this armament, primary care physicians are well-equipped to diagnose and treat patients with GBD.

ACKNOWLEDGMENT

The authors thank Dr. Kandace Klein (Assistant Professor, Department of Radiology and Imaging, Medical College of Georgia at Augusta University) for selection of all radiology images used in the article. They acknowledge her expertise and guidance.

REFERENCES

1. Everhart JE, Khare M, Hill M, et al. Prevalence and ethnic differences in gallbladder disease in the United States. Gastroenterology 1999;117(3):632–9.
2. Sandler RS, Everhart JE, Donowitz M, et al. The burden of selected digestive diseases in the United States. Gastroenterology 2002;122(5):1500–11.
3. Chen W, Mo JJ, Lin L, et al. Diagnostic value of magnetic resonance cholangiopancreatography in choledocholithiasis. World J Gastroenterol 2015;21(11): 3351–60.
4. Portincasa P, Moschetta A, Palasciano G. Cholesterol gallstone disease. Lancet 2006;368(9531):230–9.
5. Diehl AK. Epidemiology and natural history of gallstone disease. Gastroenterol Clin North Am 1991;20(1):1–19.
6. Heaton KW, Braddon FE, Mountford RA, et al. Symptomatic and silent gall stones in the community. Gut 1991;32(3):316–20.
7. Friedman GD. Natural history of asymptomatic and symptomatic gallstones. Am J Surg 1993;165(4):399–404.
8. Gibney EJ. Asymptomatic gallstones. Br J Surg 1990;77(4):368–72.
9. Kimura Y, Takada T, Kawarada Y, et al. Definitions, pathophysiology, and epidemiology of acute cholangitis and cholecystitis: Tokyo Guidelines. J Hepatobiliary Pancreat Sci 2007;(14):15–26.
10. Strasberg SM. Clinical practice. Acute calculous cholecystitis. N Engl J Med 2008;358(26):2804–11.
11. Trowbridge RL, Rutkowski NK, Shojania KG. Does this patient have acute cholecystitis? JAMA 2003;289(1):80–6.

12. Portincasa P, Moschetta A, Petruzzelli M, et al. Gallstone disease: symptoms and diagnosis of gallbladder stones. Best Pract Res Clin Gastroenterol 2006;20(6): 1017–29.

13. Yarmish GM, Smith MP, Rosen MP, et al. ACR appropriateness criteria right upper quadrant pain. J Am Coll Radiol 2014;11(3):316–22.

14. Kiewiet JJ, Leeuwenburgh MM, Bipat S, et al. A systematic review and meta-analysis of diagnostic performance of imaging in acute cholecystitis. Radiology 2012;264(3):708–20.

15. Katabathina VS, Zafar AM, Suri R. Clinical presentation, imaging, and management of acute cholecystitis. Tech Vasc Interv Radiol 2015;18(4):256–65.

16. Akriviadis EA, Hatzigavriel M, Kapnias D, et al. Treatment of biliary colic with diclofenac: a randomized, double-blind, placebo-controlled study. Gastroenterology 1997;113(1):225–31.

17. Henderson SO, Swadron S, Newton E. Comparison of intravenous ketorolac and meperidine in the treatment of biliary colic. J Emerg Med 2002;23(3):237–41.

18. Thomas SH, Silen W. Effect on diagnostic efficiency of analgesia for undifferentiated abdominal pain. Br J Surg 2003;90(1):5–9.

19. Venneman NG, Besselink MG, Keulemans YC, et al. Ursodeoxycholic acid exerts no beneficial effect in patients with symptomatic gallstones awaiting cholecystectomy. Hepatology 2006;43(6):1276–83.

20. Zafar SN, Obirieze A, Adesibikan B, et al. Optimal time for early laparoscopic cholecystectomy for acute cholecystitis. JAMA Surg 2015;150(2):129–36.

21. Hirota M, Takada T, Kawarada Y, et al. Diagnostic criteria and severity assessment of acute cholecystitis: Tokyo Guidelines. J Hepatobiliary Pancreat Surg 2007;14(1):78–82.

22. Gurusamy KS, Davidson C, Gluud C, et al. Early versus delayed laparoscopic cholecystectomy for people with acute cholecystitis. Cochrane Database Syst Rev 2013;(6):CD005440.

23. Keus F, de Jong JA, Gooszen HG, et al. Laparoscopic versus open cholecystectomy for patients with symptomatic cholecystolithiasis. Cochrane Database Syst Rev 2006;(4):CD006231.

24. Simorov A, Ranade A, Parcells J, et al. Emergent cholecystostomy is superior to open cholecystectomy in extremely ill patients with acalculous cholecystitis: a large multicenter outcome study. Am J Surg 2013;206(6):935–40 [discussion: 940–1].

25. Williams EJ, Green J, Beckingham I, et al. Guidelines on the management of common bile duct stones (CBDS). Gut 2008;57(7):1004–21.

26. Copelan A, Kapoor BS. Choledocholithiasis: diagnosis and management. Tech Vasc Interv Radiol 2015;18(4):244–55.

27. Park SM, Kim WS, Bae IH, et al. Common bile duct dilatation after cholecystectomy: a one-year prospective study. J Korean Surg Soc 2012;83(2):97–101.

28. Choi BI, Han JK, Hong ST, et al. Clonorchiasis and cholangiocarcinoma: etiologic relationship and imaging diagnosis. Clin Microbiol Rev 2004;17(3):540–52. Table of contents.

29. Caddy GR, Tham TC. Gallstone disease: symptoms, diagnosis and endoscopic management of common bile duct stones. Best Pract Res Clin Gastroenterol 2006;20(6):1085–101.

30. Sethi S, Wang F, Korson AS, et al. Prospective assessment of consensus criteria for evaluation of patients with suspected choledocholithiasis. Dig Endosc 2016; 28(1):75–82.

31. Gurusamy KS, Giljaca V, Takwoingi Y, et al. Ultrasound versus liver function tests for diagnosis of common bile duct stones. Cochrane Database Syst Rev 2015;(2):CD011548.

32. Ansaloni L, Pisano M, Coccolini F, et al. 2016 WSES guidelines on acute calculous cholecystitis. World J Emerg Surg 2016;11:25.

33. Stott MA, Farrands PA, Guyer PB, et al. Ultrasound of the common bile duct in patients undergoing cholecystectomy. J Clin Ultrasound 1991;19(2):73–6.

34. ASGE Standards of Practice Committee, Maple JT, Ben-Menachem T, Anderson MA, et al. The role of endoscopy in the evaluation of suspected choledocholithiasis. Gastrointest Endosc 2010;71(1):1–9.

35. Tseng CW, Chen CC, Chen TS, et al. Can computed tomography with coronal reconstruction improve the diagnosis of choledocholithiasis? J Gastroenterol Hepatol 2008;23(10):1586–9.

36. Kaltenthaler E, Vergel YB, Chilcott J, et al. A systematic review and economic evaluation of magnetic resonance cholangiopancreatography compared with diagnostic endoscopic retrograde cholangiopancreatography. Health Technol Assess 2004;8(10):iii, 1–89.

37. Tse F, Liu L, Barkun AN, et al. EUS: a meta-analysis of test performance in suspected choledocholithiasis. Gastrointest Endosc 2008;67(2):235–44.

38. Gurusamy KS, Giljaca V, Takwoingi Y, et al. Endoscopic retrograde cholangiopancreatography versus intraoperative cholangiography for diagnosis of common bile duct stones. Cochrane Database Syst Rev 2015;(2):CD010339.

39. Machi J, Oishi AJ, Tajiri T, et al. Routine laparoscopic ultrasound can significantly reduce the need for selective intraoperative cholangiography during cholecystectomy. Surg Endosc 2007;21(2):270–4.

40. Ahmed S, Schlachter TR, Hong K. Percutaneous transhepatic cholangioscopy. Tech Vasc Interv Radiol 2015;18(4):201–9.

41. Giljaca V, Gurusamy KS, Takwoingi Y, et al. Endoscopic ultrasound versus magnetic resonance cholangiopancreatography for common bile duct stones. Cochrane Database Syst Rev 2015;(2). CD011549. Available at: http://onlinelibrary.wiley.com/doi/10.1002/14651858.CD011549/abstract.

42. Brand M, Bizos D, Peter J, et al. Antibiotic prophylaxis for patients undergoing elective endoscopic retrograde cholangiopancreatography. Cochrane Database Syst Rev 2010;(10):CD007345.

43. Oh HC, Lee SK, Lee TY, et al. Analysis of percutaneous transhepatic cholangioscopy-related complications and the risk factors for those complications. Endoscopy 2007;39(8):731–6.

44. Prasson P, Bai X, Zhang Q, et al. One-stage laproendoscopic procedure versus two-stage procedure in the management for gallstone disease and biliary duct calculi: a systemic review and meta-analysis. Surg Endosc 2016;30(8):3582–90.

45. Shen F, Pawlik TM. Surgical management of choledocholithiasis: a disappearing skill. JAMA Surg 2016;151(12):1130–1.

46. Boey J, Way L. Acute cholangitis. Ann Surg 1980;(191):264.

47. Kiriyama S, Takada T, Strasberg SM, et al. New diagnostic criteria and severity assessment of acute cholangitis in revised Tokyo Guidelines. J Hepatobiliary Pancreat Sci 2012;19(5):548–56.

48. Gomi H, Solomkin JS, Takada H, et al. TG13 Antimicrobial therapy for acute cholangitis and cholecystitis. J Hepatobiliary Pancreat Surg 2013;(20):60–70.

49. Kimura Y, Takada T, Strasberg SM, et al. TG13 current terminology, etiology, and epidemiology of acute cholangitis and cholecystitis. J Hepatobiliary Pancreat Sci 2013;20(1):8–23.

50. Mosler P. Diagnosis and management of acute cholangitis. Curr Gastroenterol Rep 2011;13:166–72.
51. Rosing DK, DeVirgilio C, Nguyen AT, et al. Cholangitis: analysis of admission prognostic indicators and outcomes. Am Surg 2007;73:949–54.
52. Kiriyama S, Takada T, Strasberg SM, et al. TG13 guidelines for diagnosis and severity grading of acute cholangitis (with videos). J Hepatobiliary Pancreat Sci 2013;20(1):24–34.
53. Tanaka A, Takada T, Kawarada Y, et al. Antimicrobial therapy for acute cholangitis: Tokyo Guidelines. J Hepatobiliary Pancreat Surg 2007;14(1):59–67.
54. Miura F, Takada T, Kawarada Y, et al. Flowcharts for the diagnosis and treatment of acute cholangitis and cholecystitis: Tokyo Guidelines. J Hepatobiliary Pancreat Surg 2007;14(1):27–34.
55. Akcakaya A, Koc B, Adas G, et al. The use of ERCP during pregnancy: is it safe and effective? Hepatogastroenterol 2014;61(130):296–8.
56. Shaffer E. Acalculous biliary pain: new concepts for an old entity. Dig Liver Dis 2003;35(Suppl 3):S20–5.
57. Croteau DI. Speed your diagnosis of this gallbladder disorder. J Fam Pract 2013; 62(1):4–8.
58. Al-Azzawi HH, Nakeeb A, Saxena R, et al. Cholecystosteatosis: an explanation for increased cholecystectomy rates. J Gastrointest Surg 2007;11(7):835–42 [discussion: 842–3].
59. Drossman DA, Li Z, Andruzzi E, et al. U.S. householder survey of functional gastrointestinal disorders. Prevalence, sociodemography, and health impact. Dig Dis Sci 1993;38(9):1569–80.
60. Goldblatt MI, Swartz-Basile DA, Al-Azzawi HH, et al. Nonalcoholic Fatty gallbladder disease: the influence of diet in lean and obese mice. J Gastrointest Surg 2006;10(2):193–201.
61. Cotton PB, Elta GH, Carter CR, et al. Gallbladder and sphincter of Oddi disorders. Gastroenterology 2016. [Epub ahead of print].
62. Ponsky TA, DeSagun R, Brody F. Surgical therapy for biliary dyskinesia: a meta-analysis and review of the literature. J Laparoendosc Adv Surg Tech A 2005; 15(5):439–42.
63. Sgouros SN, Pereira SP. Systematic review: sphincter of Oddi dysfunction–noninvasive diagnostic methods and long-term outcome after endoscopic sphincterotomy. Aliment Pharmacol Ther 2006;24(2):237–46.
64. Behar J, Corazziari E, Guelrud M, et al. Functional gallbladder and sphincter of Oddi disorders. Gastroenterology 2006;130(5):1498–509.
65. Toouli J. Biliary dyskinesia. Curr Treat Options Gastroenterol 2002;5(4):285–91.
66. Bistritz L, Bain VG. Sphincter of Oddi dysfunction: managing the patient with chronic biliary pain. World J Gastroenterol 2006;12(24):3793–802.
67. Steele J, Wayne M, Iskandar M, et al. Biliary pain, no gallstones: remove the gallbladder, anyway? J Fam Pract 2014;63(8):421–3.
68. DuCoin C, Faber R, Ilagan M, et al. Normokinetic biliary dyskinesia: a novel diagnosis. Surg Endosc 2012;26(11):3088–93.
69. Carr JA, Walls J, Bryan LJ, et al. The treatment of gallbladder dyskinesia based upon symptoms: results of a 2-year, prospective, nonrandomized, concurrent cohort study. Surg Laparosc Endosc Percutan Tech 2009;19(3):222–6.

Nonalcoholic Fatty Liver Disease

Patrick H. Sweet, MD[a],*, Teresa Khoo, MD[b], Steven Nguyen, MD[b]

KEYWORDS

- Nonalcoholic fatty liver disease (NAFLD) • Nonalcoholic steatohepatitis (NASH)
- Liver disease • Metabolic disease • Dyslipidemia • Insulin resistance • Steatosis

KEY POINTS

- Nonalcoholic fatty liver disease (NAFLD) defines a condition of hepatic steatosis with or without hepatic injury.
- NAFLD is increasing in prevalence worldwide and presents a public health burden. Most patients are asymptomatic, although some present with fatigue and right upper quadrant pain.
- NAFLD is discovered incidentally when patients have elevated liver enzymes or fatty liver is seen on imaging modalities.
- Imaging studies can confirm fatty deposits in the liver, but needle biopsy is needed to determine degree of inflammation.
- The mainstay of treatment is weight loss and controlling diabetes and hyperlipidemia; liver transplantation is considered when disease progresses to cirrhosis.

DESCRIPTION

Nonalcoholic fatty liver disease (NAFLD) describes a condition of fatty infiltration of the liver in the absence of the other common cause of steatosis, heavy alcohol consumption, which is its own entity (ie, alcoholic liver disease). NAFLD is associated with metabolic risk factors such as diabetes mellitus, dyslipidemia, obesity, and in some cases genetic predisposition.[1,2] The clinical and histologic phenotypes of NAFLD extend from a nonalcoholic fatty liver to nonalcoholic steatohepatitis (NASH).

EPIDEMIOLOGY

NAFLD is a common liver disorder that has been gradually increasing worldwide. Prevalence of NAFLD ranges from 6.3% to 33.0%, whereas prevalence of NASH ranges

Disclosure Statement: The authors have nothing to disclose.
[a] Family Medicine, University of California, Riverside, 555 Tachevah Drive, 2E-204, Palm Springs, CA 92262, USA; [b] Family Medicine Residency in Palm Springs, University of California, Riverside, 555 Tachevah Drive, 2E-204, Palm Springs, CA 92262, USA
* Corresponding author.
E-mail address: Patrick.sweet@ucr.edu

from about 3% to 5%. NAFLD affects males more than females. Hispanics have a higher prevalence when compared with non-Hispanic Caucasians, whereas Blacks have a lower prevalence compared with both. Prevalence in Native Americans is also lower, ranging from 0.6% to 2.2%.[1–4] In Asians, however, the disease seems to manifest at a lower body mass index, and many patients do not have insulin resistance as determined by using conventional methods.[2]

DEFINITIONS

NAFLD is divided into 2 categories: nonalcoholic fatty liver and NASH. Nonalcoholic fatty liver describes hepatic steatosis without the significant inflammation that leads to hepatocellular injury or fibrosis. Nonalcoholic fatty liver is usually considered benign and reversible, with minimal risk of progression to cirrhosis or liver failure. In contrast, NASH refers to hepatic steatosis with inflammation and hepatic injury in the form of ballooning of hepatocytes and resulting cellular necrosis. Because NASH is a more severe stage of NAFLD, the risk of progression to cirrhosis, liver failure, and hepatocellular carcinoma, although rare, is higher.[3,4]

PATHOGENESIS

There is significant overlap between the pathologic processes seen in NAFLD and what is seen in alcoholic liver disease. The overlap is to such a degree that a biopsy alone is not able to specify which cause has led to the organic findings. Thus, history is very important to understanding the cause of hepatic steatosis in an undifferentiated patient. Although the 2 conditions have different pathways, they share many similarities. **Fig. 1** demonstrates where these processes overlap. Despite these findings, the treatment is significantly different and therefore attention to the patient's social history is of paramount importance. Pathogenesis can, however, have some overlap in the patient that has both processes cooccurring (eg, a patient with the metabolic syndrome who also abuses ethanol).

The pathogenesis of NAFLD is still being studied. Insulin resistance is the most widely supported key mechanism leading to hepatic steatosis and then steatohepatitis. Many support a 2-hit hypothesis for the progression of NAFLD to NASH, and ultimately, cirrhosis. The initial first hit is that fat gets deposited in hepatocytes. The deposition typically occurs in a macrovesicular pattern. Most authors believe this is brought about by globally active metabolic factors, namely, insulin resistance, central obesity, and fatty acid metabolism dysregulation. The second hit is thought to be the cause of the inflammation and later fibrosis. Oxidative stress plays an important role in this second hit. The process involves induction of cytochrome P450 enzymes that

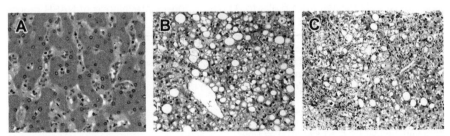

Fig. 1. Histology of (A) normal liver, (B) nonalcoholic steatosis (NAFLD), and (C) nonalcoholic steatohepatitis (NASH).

promote oxidative stress, lipid peroxidation, and mitochondrial dysfunction. It is also believed that iron deposition in the hepatocytes plays a role in the damage caused by oxidative stress. Iron deposition is thought to be a possible explanation of why men have a higher incidence of this disease than women; women have a diet lower in iron compared with men and also tend to have lower total body iron stores owing to menses.[5] These processes lead to formation of reactive oxygen species, inflammation, cell damage, and necrosis.[6–8]

Pathologically, the macrovesicular fat deposition is the initial finding (**Fig. 2**). It may be bland, appearing with no inflammation. Later in the process, a hepatocellular injury pattern known as fatty balloon degeneration occurs (see **Fig. 2**). This cellular degeneration leads to recruitment of inflammatory cells (eg, neutrophils) to the parenchyma of the organ. Inflammation then leads to repair mechanism responses that involve laying down of proteins in the intercellular matrix. This is signified by fibrosis pathologically. As this becomes advanced, the pathologic change is often described as a perisinusoidal/pericellular "chicken wire" fibrosis. When fibrosis is widespread and combined with hepatocellular cell loss, physiologic dysfunction of the organ (hepatic insufficiency) results. The degree of inflammation eventually decreases as fibrosis progresses and fewer hepatocytes are available to be injured or destroyed. The end stage of this process is cirrhosis and, as some authors have labeled, burnout NASH.[9,10]

RISK FACTORS

Risk factors associated with NAFLD are listed in **Table 1**.

CLINICAL PRESENTATION

Most patients with NAFLD are asymptomatic. Some patients may complain of nonspecific symptoms like malaise, fatigue, and vague right upper quadrant abdominal pain

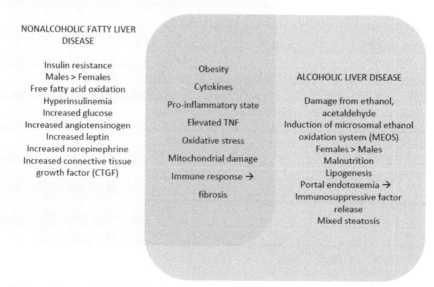

Fig. 2. Venn diagram highlighting the similarities and differences between the pathogenesis of nonalcoholic fatty liver disease and alcoholic liver disease.

Table 1
Risk factors of NAFLD and factors associated with disease progression or advanced fibrosis

Risk Factors Associated with NAFLD	Factors Associated with Disease Progression or Advanced Fibrosis
Diabetes mellitus	Older age
Dyslipidemia	Diabetes mellitus
Obesity	Elevated serum aminotransferases (≥ 2 times the upper limit of normal)
Metabolic syndrome	Presence of ballooning degeneration and Mallory hyaline or fibrosis on biopsy
Males	BMI ≥ 28 kg/m^2

Abbreviations: BMI, body mass index; NAFLD, nonalcoholic fatty liver disease.

(**Table 2**). The most common clinical feature of NAFLD is usually central obesity. Hepatomegaly can be seen in patients with fatty infiltration of the liver. Patients with NAFLD-associated cirrhosis may have ascites or symptoms of portal hypertension.[11,12]

MAKING THE DIAGNOSIS

The diagnosis of NAFLD requires confirmation of steatosis by imaging or histology in the absence significant alcohol use, and the exclusion of other causes of steatosis and chronic liver disease. Other causes of liver disease include viral hepatitis, hemochromatosis, Wilson's disease, autoimmune disease, and iatrogenic liver damage. Diagnosis is typically suggested in asymptomatic patients based on incidental findings of elevated liver enzymes on screening laboratory tests, prompting further imaging to evaluate for the presence of steatosis or fibrosis.[13] Acquisition of histologic samples

Table 2
Signs/symptoms and laboratory associated with NAFLD

Signs/Symptoms	NAFLD	Steatohepatitis	Cirrhosis
Asymptomatic	Present	Present	Portal hypertension
Hepatomegaly	Strongly correlates	Strongly correlates	Present
Right upper quadrant pain	Strongly correlates	Strongly correlates	Present
Fever	Absent	Absent	Absent
Ascites	Absent	Absent	Present (late finding)
Jaundice	Absent	Absent	Absent
Transaminase (AST, ALT)	Normal or elevated	Normal or elevated	Normal
AST:ALT ratio	<1	<1	≥ 1
ALP	Normal or elevated	Normal or elevated	Normal
Elevated bilirubin	Absent	Absent	Absent
Thrombocytopenia	Absent	Absent	Present (late finding)
Ferritin	Normal or elevated	Normal or elevated	Normal or elevated

Abbreviations: ALP, alkaline phosphatase; ALT, alanine aminotransferase; AST, aspartate aminotransferase; NAFLD, nonalcoholic fatty liver disease.
Adapted from Brunt EM, Tiniakos DG. Fatty liver disease. In: Odze RD, Goldblum JR, editors. Surgical pathology of the GI tract, liver, biliary tract, and pancreas. 2nd edition. Philadelphia: Saunders Elsevier; 2009; with permission.

by biopsy is controversial in early stages of the disease, but is warranted in later stages to determine the severity of liver damage based on pathologic grade or stage, which can affect the treatment course.[1] Recent studies evaluating sensitivity and specificity of elastography show promise but have yet to be validated as widely as they have for other hepatitides.[10]

Clinical Laboratory Parameters

Although abnormal serum transaminases and ferritin levels are often abnormal in NAFLD, blood tests are insufficient for diagnosis of NAFLD, because they may be normal in the presence of NAFLD.[5] Laboratory testing is most important for excluding other etiologies of hepatic steatosis. In the early stages of disease, aspartate amino-transferase and ALT are the most common abnormalities, with both elevated in a ratio of aspartate aminotransferase/alanine aminotransferase ratio of less than 1. Alkaline phosphatase, gamma-glutamyltransferase, and triglycerides may also be elevated. Tests of liver function (serum bilirubin, albumin, partial thromboplastin time) are typically within normal limits if the disease has not progressed to the stages of fibrosis or cirrhosis.[14,15] Further testing should be directed at ruling out other causes, and can include fasting blood glucose, insulin sensitivity testing, and hepatitis B and C serologies. Additionally, it is useful to check a complete blood count and iron studies, in consideration of hemochromatosis, as well as a ceruloplasmin and alpha-antitrypsin A1. When multiple confirmatory tests suggest a mixed picture, autoimmune hepatitis should also be excluded.[1]

The Fibro Sure Score is calculated using 6 biomarkers (α2-macroglobulin, γ-glutanyl transpeptidase, total bilirubin, haptoglobin, apolipoprotein A1, and alanine amino-transferase), age, and gender to detect the degree of fibrosis. Studies have shown sensitivities to range between 25% and 95% and specificities from 69% to 99% with varying thresholds. According to the National Institute for Health and Care Excellence in 2016, Fibro Sure had a very serious risk of bias, serious inconsistency, and very serious imprecision.[16]

Radiologic Modalities

Imaging should be obtained when biochemical markers are elevated, and can establish the presence of hepatic steatosis, as well as rule out biliary disease or focal hepatic disease that may cause elevated liver transaminase levels. Useful studies include ultrasonography, compute tomography (CT) scans, and MRI.

Ultrasound examination is considered the first line imaging study, owing to increased sensitivity over CT scans and reduced cost. On ultrasound imaging, steatotic liver change can be visualized as hyperechogenicity of the liver owing to pockets of lipids, blurring of vascular margins, and parenchymal heterogeneity. Ultrasound imaging is not accurate in the quantification of fatty change, and has only been shown to be consistent in stratifying disease as mild or severe.[17–19]

CT scanning has increased specificity for identifying other causes of liver disease, but is not first line for determining fatty liver change, because it is more expensive than ultrasound imaging. Hepatic steatosis identified on a CT scan is usually the result of incidental detection on a CT scan ordered for other reasons.[13]

MRI is the most accurate in detecting and quantifying fatty liver change; but, like other imaging modalities, it is limited by the inability to differentiate between fatty liver, steatohepatitis, and steatohepatitis with fibrosis until very late stages of fibrotic damage or even cirrhosis.[20]

Anatomic Pathology: Needle Core Biopsy

Currently, only liver biopsy carries the sensitivity to accurately differentiate between NAFLD, NASH, and fibrosis in early stages. The role of biopsy is primarily to determine the degree of disease, namely, the extent of fibrosis and progression to cirrhosis. It can also be useful when the diagnosis is in question, because it can give more information as to the degree of hepatitis, the pattern of inflammation, and fibrosis. It is most useful for identification of fibrosis before fibrosis has progressed to a degree of severity to manifest clinical consequences, such as portal hypertension. Biopsy should be considered in patients more likely to have advanced liver disease, indicated by comorbidities such as diabetes, morbid obesity, advanced age, elevated serum ferritin, or those with persistent elevation of transaminases despite lifestyle modification. In those with severely advanced disease, staging aids in determining the need for liver transplantation. Although biopsy is generally safe, pain and complications can occur with the procedure and patient selection should be considered carefully.[1,5,12,13,17,20]

The usefulness of the liver biopsy is related to the scoring system known as the NAFLD Activity Score. Any biopsy undertaken is only useful if it can guide treatment and in this case the differentiation between NAFLD and NASH is the primary objective of biopsy. Accordingly, NAFLD Activity Score is the sum of the separate scores for steatosis (0–3), hepatocellular ballooning (0–2), and lobular inflammation (0–3), with the majority of patients with NASH having a NAFLD Activity Score of 5 or greater. This system was developed as a tool to quantify changes in NAFLD during therapeutic trials and continues to be widely used today (see **Fig. 2**; **Table 3**).[21]

TREATMENT

The 2012 Practice Guideline from the American Gastroenterological Association, American Association for the Study of Liver Diseases, and American College of Gastroenterology recommends weight reduction as the primary treatment for NAFLD, by hypocaloric diet alone or with increased physical activity. At least 3% weight

Table 3
NAFLD activity score (NAS)

Steatosis Grade	Lobular Inflammation	Hepatocellular Ballooning	NAS (0–8) = Steatosis Grade + Inflammation Grade + Ballooning Grade
0: <5%	0: None	0: None	0: None
1: 5%–33%	1: <2 foci/200× field	1: Mild (few)	1a: Mild (delicate) zone 3 perisinusoidal fibrosis, requires Masson's trichrome stain to identify
2: 34%–66%	2: 2–4/200× field	2: Moderate to marked (many)	1b: Moderate (dense) zone 3 perisinusoidal fibrosis
3: >66%	3: >4/200× field		1c: Portal fibrosis only
			2: Zone 3 perisinusoidal fibrosis with periportal fibrosis
			3: Bridging fibrosis
			4: Fibrosis

Abbreviations: NAFLD, nonalcoholic fatty liver disease; NAS, NAFLD Activity Score.
Adapted from Kleiner DE, Brunt EM, Van Natta M, et al. Design and validation of a histological scoring system for nonalcoholic fatty liver disease. Hepatology 2005;41(6):1313–21; with permission.

reduction is recommended. Medical therapies specifically directed at NAFLD and NASH have not been well-established, and as such, medical therapies are targeted at managing comorbidities (eg, metformin for diabetes). Early research into glucagon-like peptide-1 agonists (such as liraglutide and exenatide), used in the treatment of diabetes mellitus, has shown promise in reversal of fatty liver change, although an independent mechanism beyond just treating diabetes is not yet established.[19]

The 2012 Practice Guideline recommends statin therapy to treat dyslipidemia, and indicates that statin therapy is not contraindicated in patients with elevated transaminases of up to 3 times the upper limit of normal. Because statin therapy can exacerbate transaminitis from other etiologies, it should only be undertaken after the diagnosis of NAFLD has been firmly established and other causes of hepatocellular injury have been excluded. This is an example of where a biopsy could offer decision support. Although polyunsaturated omega-3 fatty acids are recommended as first-line treatment for hypertriglyceridemia, they have not been formally recommended as specific therapy for NAFLD or NASH.[1]

Because oxidative stress plays a prominent role in the development of NAFLD, antioxidants have been suggested as NAFLD therapy. Ursodeoxycholic acid, a bile acid with cytoprotective and antioxidant activity, has shown improvement in serologic markers but have not demonstrated histologic improvement. Vitamin E, although exhibiting high antioxidant action with reduced hepatocellular ballooning, has been shown to increase all-cause mortality, and is not recommended. Silymarin, or milk thistle, is a plant-based extract with antioxidant properties, and in 1 study showed a good effect on serologic markers but is unknown to affect histologic improvement.[22]

Chronic hepatic injury increases the renin–angiotensin system response in the liver, which activates inflammatory cells and contributes to progression to fibrosis. In rodent models, angiotensin-converting-enzyme inhibitors and angiotensin receptor blockers caused a reduction in hyaluronic acid and transforming growth factor-beta (which are both serologic markers of fibrosis) and a histologic score of fibrosis. These have not been studied in humans.[23]

The gut flora has been implicated in multiple immunologic defenses in the intestine, including turnover and development of the intestinal microvilli. In patients with NASH, gut permeability is increased leading to high blood levels of bacterial endotoxins, which results in liver injury.[24] Moderation of the gut flora with probiotics has been shown to cause improvement of liver histology, fatty acid content, aspartate aminotransferase, alanine aminotransferase, gamma-glutamyltransferase, and triglycerides.

Surgical considerations for liver disease that has advanced to steatohepatitis (determined by histology or clinical sequelae) include bariatric surgery and liver transplantation for those advanced to cirrhosis. Because NAFLD can be reversed with lifestyle modification, surgical intervention is not indicated. Bariatric weight loss surgery can reduce the severity of hepatic steatosis and steatohepatitis, but is not recommended as a direct treatment option for NASH (although many believe this indirectly is therapeutic).[25] Liver transplantation is indicated in the presence of acute liver failure, cirrhosis with complications (eg, ascites, encephalopathy, liver cancer), hepatopulmonary syndrome, or portopulmonary hypertension. Transplantation is contraindicated in patients who are poor candidates to undergo surgery under general anesthesia owing to severe cardiac or pulmonary disease, have fulminant AIDS (although well-controlled human immunodeficiency virus infection is not a contraindication), are continuously abusing alcohol or illicit drugs, are persistently nonadherent to treatment (because patients will need to adhere to long-term immunosuppressive regimens after transplantation), or lacking an adequate social support system.[1]

PREVENTION AND SCREENING

Primary prevention of NAFLD is aimed at prevention of obesity and insulin resistance. This is well-achieved with diet and exercise to reduce weight and thereby reduce insulin resistance. Patients should also be encouraged to limit alcohol use to prevent the development of alcohol-induced liver disease. Those with established NAFLD should be immunized for hepatitis A and B, which both worsen liver disease. Routine screening for NAFLD is not recommended in the general population. NAFLD is usually an incidental finding of elevated hepatic enzymes or imaging pursued for other purposes.[1,26]

REFERENCES

1. Chalasani N, Younossi Z, Lavine JE, et al. The diagnosis and management of non-alcoholic fatty liver disease: practice guideline by the American Association for the Study of Liver Diseases, American College of Gastroenterology, and American Gastroenterological Association. Hepatology 2012;55(6):2005–23.
2. Loomba R, Sanyal AJ. The global NAFLD epidemic. Nat Rev Gastroenterol Hepatol 2013;10:686–90.
3. Bellentani S, Marino M. Epidemiology and natural history of non-alcoholic fatty liver disease (NAFLD). Ann Hepatol 2009;8(1):S4–8.
4. Ong JP, Younossi JM. Epidemiology and natural history of NAFLD and NASH. Clin Liver Dis 2007;11(1):1–16.
5. Shim JJ. Body iron, serum ferritin, and nonalcoholic fatty liver disease. Korean J Hepatol 2012;18(1):105–7.
6. Machado MV, Cortez-Pinto H. Non-alcoholic fatty liver disease: what the clinician needs to know. World J Gastroenterol 2014;20(36):12956–80.
7. Sharma M, Mitnala S, Vishnubhotla RK, et al. The riddle of nonalcoholic fatty liver disease: progression from nonalcoholic fatty liver to nonalcoholic steatohepatitis. J Clin Exp Hepatol 2015;5(2):147–58.
8. Lee WH, Park SY, Kim SU, et al. Discrimination of nonalcoholic steatohepatitis using transient elastography in patients with nonalcoholic fatty liver disease. PLoS One 2016;11(6):e0156358.
9. Takahashi Y, Fukusato T. Histopathology of nonalcoholic fatty liver disease/nonalcoholic steatohepatitis. World J Gastroenterol 2014;20(42):15539–48.
10. Magee N, Zou A, Zhang Y. Pathogenesis of nonalcoholic steatohepatitis: interactions between liver parenchymal and nonparenchymal cells. Biomed Res Int 2016;2016:1–11.
11. Abd El-Kader SM, El-Den Ashmawy EM. Non-alcoholic fatty liver disease: the diagnosis and management. World J Hepatol 2015;7(6):846–58.
12. Brunt EM, Tiniakos DG. Fatty liver disease. In: Odze RD, Goldblum JR, editors. Surgical pathology of the GI tract, liver, biliary tract, and pancreas. 2nd edition. Philadelphia: Saunders Elsevier; 2009.
13. Bayard M, Holt J, Boroughs E. Nonalcoholic fatty liver disease. Am Fam Physician 2006;73(11):1961–8.
14. Mofrad P, Contos MJ, Haque M, et al. Clinical and histologic spectrum of nonalcoholic fatty liver disease associated with normal ALT values. Hepatology 2003;37(6):1286.
15. Charatcharoenwitthaya P, Lindor KD, Angulo P. The spontaneous course of liver enzymes and its correlation in nonalcoholic fatty liver disease. Dig Dis Sci 2012;57(7):1925–31.

16. National Institute for Health and Care Excellence. Non-alcoholic fatty liver disease: assessment and management. London: National Guideline Centre (UK); 2016.
17. Farrell GC, Larter CZ. Nonalcoholic fatty liver disease: from steatosis to cirrhosis. Hepatology 2006;43(2 Suppl 1):S99–112.
18. Sanyal AJ. AGA technical review on nonalcoholic fatty liver disease. Gastroenterology 2002;123(5):1705–25.
19. Liu J, Wang G, Jia Y, et al. GLP-1 receptor agonists: effects on the progression of non-alcoholic fatty liver disease. Diabetes Metab Res Rev 2015;31(4):329–35.
20. Lall CG, Aisen AM, Bansal N, et al. Nonalcoholic fatty liver disease. AJR Am J Roentgenol 2008;190(4):993–1002.
21. Kleiner DE, Brunt EM, Van Natta M, et al. Design and validation of a histological scoring system for nonalcoholic fatty liver disease. Hepatology 2005;41(6):1313–21.
22. Raziel A, Sakran N, Szold A, et al. Current solutions for obesity-related liver disorders: non-alcoholic fatty liver disease and non-alcoholic steatohepatitis. Isr Med Assoc J 2015;17(4):234–8.
23. Beaton MD. Current treatment options for nonalcoholic fatty liver disease and nonalcoholic steatohepatitis. Can J Gastroenterol 2012;26(6):353–8.
24. Miele L, Valenza V, La Torre G, et al. Increased permeability and tight junction alterations in nonalcoholic fatty liver disease. Hepatology 2009;49(6):1877–87.
25. Rabl C, Campos GM. The impact of bariatric surgery on nonalcoholic steatohepatitis. Semin Liver Dis 2012;32(1):80–91.
26. Wilkins T, Tadkod A, Hepburn I, et al. Nonalcoholic fatty liver disease: diagnosis and management. Am Fam Physician 2013;88(1):35–42.

Pancreatitis and Pancreatic Cancer

Anne Walling, MB, ChB[a],*, Robert Freelove, MD[b]

KEYWORDS

- Acute pancreatitis • Chronic pancreatitis • Pancreatic cancer

KEY POINTS

- Acute pancreatitis is diagnosed on clinical features, serum amylase and/or lipase greater than 3 times upper limit of normal, and transabdominal ultrasound findings.
- Acute pancreatitis requires early aggressive hydration, pain control, supportive care, management of complications, and prevention of recurrence. About 80% of cases recover spontaneously within a few days. Early cholecystectomy is indicated for gallstone-associated cases.
- In chronic pancreatitis, extensive gland destruction results in debilitating pain and symptoms of exocrine and endocrine dysfunction, including steatorrhea, malabsorption, fat-soluble vitamin deficiency, osteoporosis, and diabetes.
- Progression to chronic pancreatitis, and possibly pancreatic cancer, depends on a combination of genetic predisposition and risk factors, especially alcohol use and smoking.

Multiple risk factors exist for pancreatic cancer, including chronic pancreatitis (CP), diabetes mellitus, cigarette smoking, obesity and physical inactivity, family history of pancreatic cancer, and several inherited cancer syndromes. Five-year survival after diagnosis is extremely low (8%) because most pancreatic cancers are discovered at an advanced stage. Nevertheless, routine screening of asymptomatic adults is not recommended at this time. Common presenting signs and symptoms include jaundice, vague abdominal pain, weight loss, and hepatomegaly. Laboratory findings can further suggest pancreatic cancer, but diagnosis is made through abdominal imaging: ultrasound (US), computed tomography (CT) scan, or endoscopic US (EUS).

The authors have nothing to disclose.
[a] Department of Family and Community Medicine, University of Kansas School of Medicine-Wichita, 1010 North Kansas, Wichita, KS 67214, USA; [b] Department of Family and Community Medicine, University of Kansas School of Medicine-Wichita, Smoky Hill Family Medicine Residency, 651 East Prescott Avenue, Salina, KS 67401, USA
* Corresponding author.
E-mail address: awalling@kumc.edu

http://dx.doi.org/10.1016/j.pop.2017.07.004
0095-4543/17/   **primarycare.theclinics.com**

Surgical resection can improve 5-year survival but less than half of patients are candidates for resection at the time of diagnosis. A standard chemotherapy regimen has not yet been established and enrollment in a clinical trial is preferred for patients with unresectable tumors. Pain, jaundice, nausea, and vomiting can be severe in patients with pancreatic cancer. It is recommended that palliative care teams be involved early in treatment. Patients should also be considered for hospice as early as appropriate to maximize hospice benefit and end-of-life comfort.

ACUTE PANCREATITIS

Acute pancreatitis (AP) ranges in severity from mild inflammation to severe pancreatic necrosis, systemic inflammatory response, and organ failure.[1] About 80% of cases recover spontaneously within a few days. Annually in the United States, AP is responsible for 275,000 hospital admissions, 1,300,000 bed days, 330,500 emergency department visits, and 410,000 ambulatory consultations. Hospitalizations have increased by 38% since 2003. Health care costs are estimated at more than $2.5 billion.[2]

The annual incidence is 13 to 45 per 100,000 population. Women and men are equally affected but rates are significantly higher in blacks. Rising rates are attributed to the aging population, increases in risk factors, and improved diagnostic testing.[3]

Causes and Risk Factors

Gallstones are believed to cause 40% to 70%, and alcohol 25% to 35%, of AP cases (**Table 1**).[1,4] Rare causes include endoscopic retrograde cholangiopancreatography (ERCP), medications (eg, valproate, steroids, azathioprine), hypertriglyceridemia, infection (eg, mumps, coxsackie B4), abdominal trauma, or pancreatic structural abnormalities.[1,4–6] Pancreatic tumor should be considered in patients older than 40 years and genetic causes in those younger than 30 years of age if other risk factors are not present.[4] Abdominal obesity (waist circumference >105 cm) doubles the risk of AP

Table 1 Acute pancreatitis: factors associated with progression to a severe course	
Patient factors	Age >56 y Body mass index >30 kg/m^2 Comorbid health conditions
Signs of systemic inflammatory response syndrome (SIRS)[a]	Tachycardia (>90 beats/min) Tachypnea (>20 breaths/min) Elevated or decreased temperature (>38°C or <36°C) Elevated or suppressed WBC (>12,000 or <4000 WBC/mm^2) Altered mental status
Signs of hypovolemia[a]	Elevated or rising BUN (>20 mg/dL) Elevated or rising HCT (>44%) Elevated or rising creatinine
Imaging evidence of organ damage[a]	Pleural effusions or infiltrates Extrapancreatic fluid collections Pancreatic necrosis

Abbreviations: BUN, blood urea nitrogen; WBC, white blood count.
  [a] At presentation or developing within 24 to 48 h of hospital admission.
Data from Refs.[1,4–6]

and high body mass index is associated with increased severity and mortality.[3] Type 2 diabetes is an independent risk factor, especially for patients younger than 45 years. Smoking doubles the risk for nongallstone AP.[3]

Diagnosis

The typical presentation is severe, constant pain in the epigastrium or left upper abdomen that may radiate to the back, flanks, or chest. Patients commonly report nausea and/or vomiting, indigestion, or abdominal fullness. History and physical examination findings depend on the severity. Presentation ranges from mild symptoms and relatively normal physical examination to severe pain and symptoms of peritonitis and shock. Diagnosis requires at least 2 criteria out of (1) characteristic pain, (2) serum amylase and/or lipase greater than 3 times upper limit of normal, and (3) characteristic findings on abdominal imaging.[4]

Enzyme testing

Serum amylase increases within hours of symptom onset and remains elevated for 3 to 5 days. Serum lipase remains elevated longer and is more specific than amylase. False-negative enzyme levels are common, especially in alcoholism or hypertriglyceridemia. False-positive elevations may occur in renal and salivary gland conditions, as well as other abdominal inflammations. For unknown reasons, diabetic patients have high median lipase levels, so the upper limit of normal for lipase is 3 to 5 times higher in diabetic patients.[4] Because of test accuracy concerns, guidelines stress imaging in patients with clinical features of AP even if enzyme levels are not elevated.[4]

Imaging

Transabdominal US is recommended for all patients with AP.[4] MRI or contrast-enhanced CT (CECT) is indicated if the diagnosis is uncertain or if the patient fails to improve within 48 to 72 hours of treatment. Both CECT and MRI have greater than 90% sensitivity and specificity for the diagnosis of AP, but MRI can also identify gall stones greater than 3 mm diameter. ERCP is only indicated in AP patients with concurrent cholangitis.[4]

Classification and triage

Scoring systems to predict which patients will progress to severe disease have high false-positive rates and typically require 48 hours to become accurate. By then, severity is usually clinically obvious.[4] Guidelines recommend individualized assessment of risk for progression to systemic inflammatory response syndrome (SIRS) and organ failure based on clinical, laboratory, and imaging findings rather than formal scoring systems[4] (see **Table 1**).

Management

Management of AP requires diligent monitoring, supportive care, early aggressive hydration, pain control, management of complications, and prevention of recurrence and progression to CP.

Monitoring

Monitoring is essential for the first 48 to 72 hours of symptoms. Patients at risk of severe AP (**Table 2**) should be managed in intensive care units. In addition to vital signs, urine output and oxygen saturation should be monitored every 1 to 2 hours and physical examination repeated every 4 to 8 hours. Laboratory values, including blood counts, calcium, glucose, magnesium, and blood urea nitrogen (BUN), should be checked every 6 to 12 hours.[5] Imaging should be performed for indications of

Table 2	
Cause of pancreatitis	
Acute	**Chronic**
Gallstones or other biliary obstruction (40%–59%)	Alcohol (50%)
Alcohol (25%–30%)	Tobacco
Hypertriglyceridemia (>1,000 mg/dl)	Recurrent, severe AP
Medication	Genetic
ERCP	Obstructive
Autoimmune	Chronic renal failure
Genetic (including cystic fibrosis)	Hyperparathyroidism
Idiopathic (10%–30%)	Toxins or drugs

Patient may have multiple, synergistic risk factors.
Data from Refs.[1,4–7]

developing complications such as pancreatic necrosis. Noninvasive modalities are preferred, but early ERCP may be beneficial in patients with biliary sepsis.[4] Physicians must be prepared to respond quickly to developing complications and to promptly transfer patients with AP to higher levels of care if indicated.

Early aggressive intravenous hydration

The cornerstone of AP management is aggressive early intravenous fluid resuscitation. This aims to prevent microangiopathic changes and hypovolemia that initiate the pathologic cascade, leading to organ failure. Isotonic crystalloid solution (preferably lactated Ringer solution) should be provided at 250 to 500 mL per hour during the first 12 to 24 hours and as needed thereafter. Aggressive fluid administration for more than 24 hours has little evidence of benefit. The BUN can be used to monitor fluid requirements. More aggressive fluid repletion may be indicated in hypovolemic patients. Conversely, less aggressive therapy and more careful monitoring is indicated for elderly patients and those with cardiac conditions, renal disease, or other risk of overload.[1,4–6,8]

Nutrition

Previously, patients were nil by mouth (npo) until pain reduction and/or improvement in enzyme levels. Current guidelines recommend oral low-fat, low-residue soft diet for mild AP as soon as improvement is evident. Soft diet provides more calories and may reduce hospital stay compared with liquid diet.[4,8] In more severe cases, enteral nutrition by nasogastric or nasojejunal delivery is recommended to support the gut mucosal barrier and reduce infectious complications. Total parenteral nutrition should be avoided.[4]

Medications

No analgesic seems to have specific efficacy in AP. Opiates are frequently used.[6] Antiemetics and other agents may alleviate symptoms. The role of antibiotics is controversial. Early antibiotic therapy does not reduce rates of infection, infected necrotizing pancreatitis, or mortality.[4,6] Current guidelines recommend against routine prophylactic antibiotics, even in severe AP, but support targeted antibiotic use for extrapancreatic infections or infected pancreatic necrosis. The selection of antibiotic must be driven by culture results. For infected pancreatic necrosis, agents must penetrate the target tissue (carbapenems, quinolones, metronidazole, high-dose cephalosporins). Probiotics provide no benefit in severe AP and may increase mortality.[4–6]

Surgical Treatment

Patients hospitalized for mild gallstone-associated AP should undergo cholecystectomy before discharge.[4] Strong evidence is lacking to guide decisions regarding the optimal timing of surgery in severe AP, including pancreatic necrosis.[4,9]

Follow-up

Patients may require support for anorexia, weight loss, and deconditioning following severe AP. The need for enzyme supplements is unclear.[6] Risk factors, such as alcohol use, smoking, hypertriglyceridemia, and obesity, should be addressed.

Outcomes

The overall mortality of AP is about 1% to 2% but increases with age, comorbidities, and severity. Mortality reaches more than 30% in patients with hemorrhagic or necrotizing pancreatitis, pancreatic abscess, or multiorgan dysfunction. About 20% to 30% of patients suffer recurrence and around 10% progress to CP.[3] Impaired endocrine and exocrine function persist in 20% to 30% of patients and these patients are at high risk of transitioning to CP.[1]

CHRONIC PANCREATITIS

CP is now defined as "a pathologic fibro-inflammatory syndrome of the pancreas in individuals with genetic, environmental, and/or other risk factors who develop persistent pathologic responses to parenchymal injury or stress." The definition also states, "Common features of established and advanced CP include pancreatic atrophy, fibrosis, pain syndromes, duct distortion and strictures, calcifications, pancreatic exocrine dysfunction, pancreatic endocrine dysfunction, and dysplasia."[10]

Epidemiology, Causes, and Risk Factors

The etiologic classification of CP is often as structural or obstructive (eg, stones, strictures, neoplasm), metabolic (eg, hypertriglyceridemia), infectious (eg, recurrent AP), toxic (eg, alcohol, drugs), genetic, and other.[7] A specific cause cannot be established in up to 30% of cases[11] (see **Table 2**).

Because many cases are not diagnosed, the true impact of CP is unknown. The prevalence is about 50 per 100,000 population and 5 to 12 new cases are diagnosed per 100,000 annually.[3] More than 275,000 emergency department visits for CP were documented in 2012, of which 30% required hospitalization.[2] CP is more common in men and in blacks. Because most cases are linked to prolonged heavy alcohol use (>150 mL/d for at least 6 years), the average age at diagnosis is 35 to 55 years; however, cases occur in children and young adults with cystic fibrosis or other genetic and/or anatomic defects.[11]

The current model describes progression from recurrent AP to early, established, and end-stage CP and stresses the interplay of injury and response in individual patients.[12] Several genetic factors have been implicated in the development of CP.[7] Progression from AP is also related to the severity of the attacks, smoking, and alcohol use.[13] After a first episode of alcohol-related AP, the risk of progression to CP is 14%

with abstinence but increases to 41% with continuation of previous alcohol intake.[3] Smoking and alcohol often coexist and are synergistic.[14] Smoking alone contributes 25% of the risk of CP and accelerates disease progression.[3]

Clinical Features

Patients usually suffer recurrent attacks of AP. The triad of chronic or recurrent pain, exocrine dysfunction, and/or diabetes indicates progression to CP.[14] Pain is the dominant symptom. It occurs in the epigastrium and/or upper quadrants, often postprandially, may radiate to the back, and be relieved by sitting upright or leaning forward. Nausea, vomiting, and weight loss are common. Patients commonly experience fatigue, sleep disturbance, anxiety, depression, and low quality of life.[12] Exocrine insufficiency is under-recognized and can cause steatorrhea, malnutrition, and deficiencies of vitamins A, D, E, K, B_{12}, thiamine, and folic acid, as well as calcium and magnesium. An estimated 40% of CP patients develop osteopenia and an additional 25% become osteoporotic.[15] Endocrine dysfunction from extensive pancreatic destruction is termed type 3 diabetes.[7,11,14]

Diagnosis

Especially if the exocrine and/or endocrine features are missed, CP may be misdiagnosed as peptic ulcer, gastritis, biliary or liver disease, renal conditions, or other causes of abdominal, flank or back pain. Diagnostic testing depends on an individualized approach to rule out other conditions and confirm chronic pancreatic changes. The accuracy of all diagnostic testing improves with advanced disease. No single test is reliably diagnostic for early CP and no evidence-based guidelines are available for diagnostic strategy.[14]

Imaging

EUS is reported to be 80% to 90% sensitive and more than 80% specific, depending on the criteria applied for CP.[14] EUS has largely replaced ERCP and is more sensitive than CT or magnetic resonance cholangiopancreatography (MRCP).[14] Advanced changes, such as calcified pancreatic ducts, pseudocysts, necrosis, and atrophy, can be detected with CT.[11,14,16]

Laboratory testing

During acute exacerbations, pancreatic enzyme levels may be elevated and elevations of hepatic enzymes and bilirubin occur in biliary obstruction.[11] The only direct pancreatic function test is endoscopic collection of fluid after stimulation with secretin. This can be combined with EUS but is rarely used and false positives are reported.[11,14,16] The most common indirect assessments of pancreatic function are fecal elastase 1 and 72-h fecal fat. Fecal fat measurements have better sensitivity and specificity but are more cumbersome to perform.[14]

Management

The goals of treatment are management of pain and exocrine and endocrine dysfunction, plus prevention of exacerbations, progression, and complications.

The severe, debilitating pain is often treated with opiates or tramadol, but CP patients have high risk of addiction and adverse effects. Increasing evidence supports central sensitization in pain severity and persistence.[12] Antidepressants and pregabalin may help relieve pain and depressive comorbidities but no guidelines are available. Lifestyle changes in diet, smoking, and alcohol use contribute to pain reduction, as well as preventing progression of CP. Cognitive-behavioral approaches seem highly relevant but have not been studied in CP.[12] Consultation with pain specialists is often indicated.

Exocrine deficiencies require enzyme replacement (initially 40,000–50,000 units lipase with each meal), plus vitamin and calcium supplementation. Frequent small meals are recommended to provide 1.0 to 1.5 g/Kg of protein, 30% to 40% calories from fat, and limited carbohydrates.[16]

Metformin is effective for hyperglycemia but may be poorly tolerated and exacerbate weight loss. Patients with diabetes due to CP have increased risk of hypoglycemia and may have lifestyles that complicate diabetes management.[14]

Surgery

Surgery is indicated for biliary or duodenal obstructions, complications such as pseudocysts or dilated pancreatic duct, and intractable pain. Pancreatic fibrosis may limit the use of endoscopic approaches. In extreme cases, partial or total pancreatectomy with autologous islet cell transplantation may be considered.[7,11,14]

Monitoring and Follow-up

CP requires managing chronic pain, avoiding exacerbating factors, and detecting and addressing multiple complications. Self-management is desirable but alcohol, chronic debilitating symptoms, and other factors make adherence very challenging for many CP patients and their families. Patients have shortened survival times but most deaths are attributed to other chronic conditions, infections, or cancer. The risk of pancreatic cancer is 13 times higher for CP patients than controls.[3]

PANCREATIC CANCER

Pancreatic cancer is the fourth leading cause of cancer-related death in men and women in the United States.[17] It is estimated that in 2017 there will be more than 53,000 new diagnoses and more than 43,000 deaths from pancreatic cancer.[17] Five-year survival for advanced-stage pancreatic cancer is only 3%. Unfortunately, most pancreatic cancers are diagnosed at an advanced stage; therefore, the current 5-year survival for all pancreatic cancer diagnoses is only 8%. Pancreatic cancer incidence is low before age 45 but increases quickly afterward. It has a slight male-to-female predominance (1.3:1) and is more common in blacks.

Cause and Risk Factors

Nonhereditary risk factors for pancreatic cancer include CP, diabetes mellitus, cigarette smoking, obesity, and physical inactivity.[18-21] Pancreatic cancer can aggregate in some families, though a genetic basis has not been identified. The risk for development of pancreatic cancer is increased in people with a family history of pancreatic cancer in a first-degree relative; the risk increases dramatically as the number of affected first-degree relatives increases.[22] When more than 1 first-degree relative with pancreatic cancer exists in a family it is known as familial pancreatic cancer.[22] Additionally, defined hereditary syndromes in which patients are at high risk for a pancreatic cancer include BRCA1 and BRCA2 gene carriers, hereditary nonpolyposis colon cancer (Lynch syndrome), familial atypical multiple mole melanoma syndrome, hereditary pancreatitis, and Peutz-Jeghers syndrome.[23] Another inherited risk factor for developing pancreatic cancer is having a non-O blood type.[24]

Screening

There is no effective screening mechanism for asymptomatic adults at average risk. The United States Preventive Services Task Force recommends against routine screening for pancreatic cancer with palpation, ultrasonography, or serologic markers.[25] Experts agree that those with significant inherited risk factors should be initially screened with either EUS or MRCP. These modalities are preferred over CT or ERCP. However, there is lack of consensus on when to initiate screening, which modality to select, and the appropriate interval for follow-up imaging or continued screening.[26]

Clinical Presentation

Jaundice, vague abdominal pain, and weight loss are the most common presenting symptoms. Other presenting symptoms include asthenia, anorexia, dark urine, nausea, back pain, diarrhea, vomiting, steatorrhea, and thrombophlebitis. The most common signs at diagnosis include jaundice and hepatomegaly. Other less common signs present at diagnosis include right upper quadrant mass, cachexia, nontender palpable distention of the gallbladder (Courvoisier sign), epigastric mass, and ascites.[27]

The presenting symptoms depend primarily on the size and location of the tumor within the pancreas, as well as the presence or absence of metastases. Approximately 70% of pancreatic cancers are located within the head of the pancreas, 25% are located in the body or tail, and less than 5% involve the entire pancreas. Pancreatic head tumors cause bile duct obstruction resulting in jaundice, steatorrhea, weight loss, and dark urine. The jaundice is predominantly characterized by increased levels of conjugated bilirubin. Tumors in the body or tail of the pancreas generally present with nonspecific findings, including unexplained weight loss, anorexia, asthenia, nausea, and dyspepsia. An atypical presentation of type 2 diabetes in a patient 50 years or older could indicate the presence of pancreatic cancer.[28]

Diagnosis and Staging

History and physical examination alone are not sufficient to diagnose pancreatic cancer. Serologic testing is the first step. A complete blood count, electrolytes, serum aminotransferases, alkaline phosphatase, bilirubin, and lipase should be done for patients presenting with jaundice and/or abdominal pain. The serum tumor marker carbohydrate antigen 19-9 (CA 19-9) has prognostic and monitoring benefit but lacks the sensitivity and specificity to be of diagnostic value.[29]

Abdominal imaging is the next step in evaluation. The imaging modality of choice is determined by presenting signs and symptoms. For patients presenting with jaundice, transabdominal US is the imaging modality of choice. A follow-up abdominal CT scan is indicated if the US is nondiagnostic or for staging purposes if a pancreatic mass is identified on US. For patients presenting with abdominal pain and weight loss, or for any patient strongly suspected of having pancreatic cancer, abdominal CT is the preferred initial imaging test. EUS-guided fine-needle aspiration is indicated for histologic diagnosis. EUS can also be used as an alternative to CT for staging purposes.[23]

Staging of pancreatic cancer is used to determine resectability; complete surgical resection is the only potentially curative treatment. Tumors are categorized along a continuum from resectable to unresectable depending on vascular involvement, invasion of adjacent organs, and the presence of distal metastases. Triphasic contrast-enhanced helical CT can provide sufficient information for staging purposes; however, EUS can be helpful for smaller tumors, local tumor (T) and node (N) staging, and predicting vascular invasion. Staging laparoscopy is reserved for patients with presumed metastasis that could not be confirmed with imaging studies.[30]

Treatment

Resectable lesions
Only 15% to 20% of patients are candidates for surgical resection. Five-year survival rates after surgical resection range from 10% to 30% and are influenced by tumor size and histology, presence of disease at resection margins, and lymph node involvement. Tumors in the head and neck of the pancreas are addressed with a pancreaticoduodenectomy (Whipple procedure). Variations in technique, including pylorus-preserving, subtotal stomach-preserving, and minimally invasive procedures, have not shown a significant difference in outcome.[30] Perioperative mortality has decreased significantly and is now less than 4%, primarily due to improved outcomes in centers where surgeons perform a higher volume of these procedures. Resectable tumors in the body and tail of the pancreas are uncommon because they are usually advanced at diagnosis. Resectable lesions are removed by distal pancreatectomy, which usually includes splenectomy. Postoperative adjuvant chemotherapy with gemcitabine or fluorouracil improves overall survival by a few months. Studies of neoadjuvant chemotherapy have not demonstrated improved survival or resectability and there is currently no role for neoadjuvant chemotherapy before surgery.[30]

Unresectable lesions
Unresectable lesions belong in 1 of 2 categories: locally advanced disease or metastatic disease. There is no curative treatment of unresectable pancreatic cancer. In these situations, treatment decisions should be based on goals of care, patient preference, psychological status, presence of support systems, symptom severity, performance status, and comorbid conditions. Patients should understand that the goal of treatment is primarily palliation, although some effect on survival may be achieved.

For locally advanced disease, initial chemotherapy is recommended, usually involving enrollment in a clinical trial. A standard, optimal chemotherapy regimen has not been established, but if a clinical trial is not available, potential options include gemcitabine monotherapy, gemcitabine combined with nab-paclitaxel, or combination chemotherapy with short-term infusional fluorouracil plus leucovorin, irinotecan, and oxaliplatin (FOLFIRINOX). Further treatment after initial chemotherapy depends on progression of disease and whether the patient becomes a potential candidate for resection.[31]

For metastatic disease, systemic chemotherapy has been shown to improve disease-related symptoms and survival when compared with best supportive care alone. Similar to locally advanced disease, enrollment in a clinical trial is preferred. However, if this is unavailable, chemotherapy guidelines exist guided by performance status, comorbidity, and serum bilirubin levels. FOLFIRINOX or gemcitabine plus nab-paclitaxel are the initial treatments of choice for patients with a good performance status and favorable or adequate comorbidity profile, respectively. Patients with poor functional status or comorbidity profile should receive gemcitabine monotherapy. Second-line therapy recommendations depend on the regimen received as first-line therapy [42].

Palliative care and complications
Early assessment of symptom burden, psychological status, and social supports should be performed in all patients with newly diagnosed pancreatic cancer. Early referral for palliative care services improves quality of life and reduces aggressive end-of-life care, including chemotherapy within 14 days of death, intensive care unit

admissions, emergency department visits, and hospitalizations near death.[32,33] Hospice referral should be considered as soon as appropriate to maximize benefit from hospice services.

Symptoms and complications that often need addressing include pain, biliary obstruction, gastric outlet obstruction, malnutrition, depression, and thromboembolic disease.

Pain from advanced pancreatic cancer can be significant and should be assessed frequently. Pain can be managed with opioid analgesics with or without adjuvant medications for neuropathic pain, radiation therapy, or celiac plexus neurolysis (CPN). CPN can be performed percutaneously, intraoperatively, or under EUS-guidance. It is a chemical ablation of the celiac plexus, which transmits the sensation of pain from the pancreas, with dehydrated 98% alcohol and seems to be more effective than pharmacologic therapy alone while avoiding opiate-related complications.[34]

Palliative options for jaundice due to biliary obstruction include placement of a biliary stent or surgical bypass with anastomosis between the gallbladder and jejunum or common bile duct and jejunum. Endoscopic placement of a metal biliary stent is the preferred treatment. The risk of surgery in debilitated patients with advanced disease is significant. As such, surgical bypass is reserved for those in whom endoscopic stent placement is not technically possible or for those found to have unresectable disease during surgical exploration.[35,36] Similarly, endoscopically placed, expandable-metal duodenal stents can relieve gastric outlet obstruction in patients with advanced disease, poor performance status, and a short life expectancy. Alternatively, surgical bypass can be achieved through laparoscopic gastrojejunostomy with better long-term outcomes and should be considered for patients whose life expectancy is greater than 2 months.[37]

Malnutrition and weight loss are common and usually multifactorial. Appropriate management of pain, gastric outlet obstruction, and biliary obstruction are important. Pancreatic exocrine insufficiency is a significant contributor and should be treated empirically with oral pancreatic enzyme replacement. Sufficient doses should be taken at the start, the middle, and end of meals. Anorexia and weight loss may also be treated with high-calorie diets and nutritional supplements. Caution should be exercised with appetite stimulants because they can increase the risk for development of thromboembolic disease.

The incidence of venous thromboembolism (VTE) is higher in pancreatic cancer than other common adenocarcinomas and patients should be educated about the signs and symptoms of VTE. Primary prophylaxis is not recommended in ambulatory patients. Hospitalized patients without risk of increased bleeding should receive prophylaxis with low-molecular-weight heparin (LMWH). Preferred treatment of patients who experience a VTE is long-term LMWH.[38]

REFERENCES

1. Forsmark CE, Vege SS, Wilcox CM. Acute pancreatitis. N Engl J Med 2016;375: 1972–81.
2. Peery AF, Crockett SD, Barritt AS, et al. Burden of gastrointestinal, liver, and pancreatic disease in the United States. Gastroenterology 2015;149:1731–41.
3. Yadav D, Lowenfels AB. The epidemiology of pancreatitis and pancreatic cancer. Gastroenterology 2013;144:1252–61.
4. Tenner S, Baillie J, De Witt J, et al. American College of Gastroenterology guideline: management of acute pancreatitis. Am J Gastroenterol 2013;018:1400–15.
5. Quinlan JD. Acute pancreatitis. Am Fam Physician 2014;90:632–9.

6. Johnson CD, Besselink MG, Carter R. Acute pancreatitis. BMJ 2014;349:g4859.
7. Callery MP, Freedman SD. A 21-year-old man with chronic pancreatitis. JAMA 2008;299:1588–94.
8. DiMagno MJ. Clinical update on fluid therapy and nutritional support in acute pancreatitis. Pancreatology 2015;15:583–8.
9. vanBaal MC, Besselink MG, Bakker OJ, et al. Timing of cholecystectomy after mild biliary pancreatitis: systematic review. Ann Surg 2010;255:890–6.
10. Whitcomb DC, Frulloni L, Garg P, et al. Chronic pancreatitis: an international draft consensus proposal for a new mechanistic definition. Pancreatology 2016;16: 218–24.
11. Nair RJ, Lawler L, Miller MR. Chronic pancreatitis. Am Fam Physician 2007;76: 1679–88.
12. Uc A, Andersen DK, Bellin MD, et al. Chronic pancreatitis in the 21st century -research challenges and opportunities. Summary of a National Institute of Diabetes and Digestive and Kidney Diseases workshop. Pancreas 2016;45: 1365–75.
13. Bertilsson S, Sward P, Kalaitzakis E. Factors that affect progression after first attack of acute pancreatitis. Clin Gastroenterol Hepatol 2015;13:1662–9.
14. Majumder S, Chari ST. Chronic pancreatitis. Lancet 2016;387:7–13.
15. Duggan SN, Smyth ND, Murphy A, et al. High prevalence of osteoporosis in patients with chronic pancreatitis; a systematic review and meta-analysis. Clin Gastroenterol Hepatol 2014;12:219–28.
16. Gupte AR, Forsmark CE. Chronic pancreatitis. Curr Opin Gastroenterol 2014;30: 500–5.
17. Siegel RL, Miller KD, Jemal A. Cancer Statistics, 2017. CA Cancer J Clin 2017; 67(1):7–30.
18. Bang UC, Benfield T, Hyldstrup L, et al. Mortality, cancer and comorbidities associated with chronic pancreatitis: a Danish nationwide matched-cohort study. Gastroenterology 2014;146(4):989–94.
19. Batabyal P, Vander Hoorn S, Christophi C, et al. Association of diabetes mellitus and pancreatic adenocarcinoma: a meta-analysis of 88 studies. Ann Surg Oncol 2014;21(7):2453–62.
20. Bosetti C, Lucenteforte E, Silverman DT, et al. Cigarette smoking and pancreatic cancer: an analysis from the International Pancreatic Cancer Case-Control Consortium. Ann Oncol 2012;23(7):1880–8.
21. Michaud DS, Giovannucci E, Willett WC, et al. Physical activity, obesity, height, and the risk of pancreatic cancer. JAMA 2001;286(8):921–9.
22. Jacobs EJ, Chanock SJ, Fuchs CS, et al. Family history of cancer and risk of pancreatic cancer: a pooled analysis from the Pancreatic Cancer Cohort Consortium. Int J Cancer 2010;127:1421–8.
23. De La Cruz MS, Young AP, Ruffin MT. Diagnosis and management of pancreatic cancer. Am Fam Physician 2014;89(8):626–32.
24. Klein AP, Lindstrom S, Mendelsohn JB, et al. An absolute risk model to identify individuals at elevated risk for pancreatic cancer in the general population. PLoS One 2013;8(9):e72311.
25. Final recommendation statement: pancreatic cancer: screening. U.S. Preventive Services Task Force; 2014. Available at: https://www.uspreventiveservicestaskforce. org/Page/Document/RecommendationStatementFinal/pancreatic-cancer-screening. Accessed January 29, 2017.

26. Canto MI, Harinck F, Hruban RH, et al. International Cancer of the Pancreas Screening (CAPS) Consortium summit on the management of patients with increased risk for familial pancreatic cancer. Gut 2013;62(3):339–47.
27. Porta M, Fabregat X, Malats N, et al. Exocrine pancreatic cancer: symptoms at presentation and their relation to tumour site and stage. Clin Transl Oncol 2005;7(5):189–97.
28. Girelli CM, Reguzzoni G, Limido E, et al. Pancreatic carcinoma: differences between patients with or without diabetes mellitus. Recenti Prog Med 1995;86(4):143–6.
29. Kim JE, Lee KT, Lee JK, et al. Clinical usefulness of carbohydrate antigen 19-9 as a screening test for pancreatic cancer in an asymptomatic population. J Gastroenterol Hepatol 2004;19(2):182–6.
30. Ryan DP, Hong TS, Bardeesy N. Pancreatic adenocarcinoma. N Engl J Med 2014;371:1039–49.
31. Balaban EP, Mangu PB, Khorana AA, et al. Locally advanced, unresectable pancreatic cancer: American society of clinical oncology clinical practice guideline. J Clin Oncol 2016;34(22):2654–68.
32. Sohal DP, Mangu PB, Khorana AA, et al. Metastatic pancreatic cancer: American Society of Clinical Oncology clinical practice guideline. J Clin Oncol 2016;34(23):2784–96.
33. Maltoni M, Scarpi E, Dall'Agata M, et al. Systematic versus on-demand early palliative care: results from a multicenter, randomized clinical trial. Eur J Cancer 2016;65:61–8.
34. Jang RW, Krzyzanowska MK, Zimmerman C, et al. Palliative care and the aggressiveness of end-of-life care in patients with advanced pancreatic cancer. J Natl Cancer Inst 2015;107(3) [pii:dju424].
35. Amr YM, Makharita MY. Neurolytic sympathectomy in the management of cancer pain-time effect: a prospective, randomized multicenter study. J Pain Symptom Manage 2014;48(5):944–56.
36. Moss AC, Morris E, Mac Mathuna P. Palliative biliary stents for obstructing pancreatic carcinoma. Cochrane Database Syst Rev 2006;(2):CD004200.
37. Jeurnink SM, Steyerberg EW, van Hooft JE, et al. Surgical gastrojejunostomy or endoscopic stent placement for the palliation of malignant gastric outlet obstructions (SUSTENT study): a multicenter randomized trial. Gastrointest Endosc 2010;71(3):490–9.
38. Lee AY, Levine MN, Baker RI, et al. Low-molecular-weight heparin versus a coumarin for the prevention of recurrent venous thromboembolism in patients with cancer. N Engl J Med 2003;349(2):146–53.

Hepatitis A and B Infections

Jennifer Thuener, MD

KEYWORDS

- Hepatitis A • Hepatitis B • Virus

KEY POINTS

- Hepatitis A causes acute viral hepatitis. The symptoms of nausea, vomiting, fatigue, and jaundice are self-limited.
- Hepatitis A infections are infrequent in the United States because of routine vaccination of children.
- Hepatitis B infrequently causes symptomatic acute viral hepatitis. When it does, it also presents with nausea, vomiting, abdominal pain, and jaundice.
- Hepatitis B can progress into chronic viral hepatitis, which increases the risk of developing cirrhosis and hepatocellular carcinoma.
- The incidence of hepatitis B infections is declining in the United States because of routine vaccination of children; however, significant morbidity and mortality from chronic hepatitis B still exist.

HISTORY

Epidemic jaundice has plagued the human race for centuries, with the first description found in writings by Hippocrates from the fifth century BC. Historically, epidemic jaundice was likely a combination of hepatitis A and B, because they could not be differentiated until the advent of modern medicine. Mass immunization against both hepatitis A and B began in the United States in the late twentieth century, which has drastically reduced the incidence of both hepatitis A and B.[1]

HEPATITIS A
Epidemiology

Hepatitis A virus (HAV) infections in the United States are very rare. The HAV vaccine became available in 1995, and since that time, incidence has decreased by 95%.[2] In 2014, there were only 1239 reported cases of HAV in the United States.[2] Accounting for underreporting and missed cases, the Centers for Disease Control and Prevention (CDC) estimates that there were likely nearly 2500 cases.

Department of Family and Community Medicine, University of Kansas School of Medicine-Wichita, 1010 North Kansas, Wichita, KS 67214, USA
E-mail address: jthuener@kumc.edu

Prim Care Clin Office Pract 44 (2017) 621–629
http://dx.doi.org/10.1016/j.pop.2017.07.005
0095-4543/17/© 2017 Elsevier Inc. All rights reserved.

Virus Description

HAV is a small, nonenveloped, RNA virus of the genus *Hepatovirus*. The virus was first isolated in 1979, and humans are its only natural host. HAV is a hardy virus; it can tolerate a pH as low as 1 as well as high heat.[3] HAV can also survive on surfaces outside of the human body for months.[3] This leads to easy transmission and explains the historic jaundice epidemics. It is also why both proper hygiene and decreasing the number of available hosts and reservoirs through vaccination are key factors to decreasing the incidence of HAV infection.

Transmission and Life Cycle

HAV undergoes fecal-oral transmission. Spread of the virus is increased by poor general hygiene, including absent or improper hand-washing after using the bathroom or changing diapers, before and during food preparation, and inadequate cleaning of bathroom and food preparation surfaces. The virus can be killed during proper cooking, but if food is not cooked thoroughly, or is contaminated after it is cooked, the virus can still be transmitted. In order to kill the virus, food must be heated to at least 185°F for 1 minute.[3–5] Once inside the body, it can survive in the stomach because of its tolerance of low pH. Virions reach the liver through the portal circulation and replicate inside hepatocytes. The virus is then released into the bile ducts and enters the enterohepatic cycle until it is neutralized by antibodies.[4]

Risk Factors

HAV vaccine is a part of the standard childhood vaccination series recommended for all children in the United States. Since its mass implementation in 1995, the incidence of HAV transmission as drastically decreased, greatly lowering the overall risk for HAV in the United States. However, there are still many unvaccinated adults, and several situations increase the risk of contracting HAV. These situations include living in or traveling to areas with poor sanitation, household contact with persons with HAV, sexual contact with persons with HAV, and men who have sex with men.[2,6] Any unvaccinated person with these high-risk behaviors should be vaccinated and educated on other risk reduction strategies.[2]

Incubation Period

The time from exposure to onset of symptoms ranges from 15 to 50 days, with an average of 28 days.[3,4] Viral shedding in the stool can occur during the incubation period, as early as 2 weeks before the onset of symptoms.[4] This time period is a time of increased risk of transmission because the patient does not yet know they are ill, and hand hygiene may be lax. The patient continues to shed the virus throughout the symptomatic period, and most viral shedding in the stool ends when clinical symptoms resolve. Interestingly, viral shedding in infants can continue for up to 5 months after clinical illness has resolved.[3] Infants require caregiver support in hygiene and diaper changing, making this a significant potential source of transmission.

Clinical Illness

After a variable but highly contagious incubation period, patients enter the clinical stage of the disease. Symptoms of HAV infection are nonspecific and variable and can include fatigue, fever, nausea, vomiting, anorexia, abdominal pain, and jaundice.[2–4] Illness severity ranges from asymptomatic to fulminant liver failure. Asymptomatic HAV is seen more commonly in infants and young children. Adults are more likely to experience symptoms, including jaundice. More than 70% of adult cases demonstrate jaundice during the clinical phase.[3,4] Nevertheless, fulminant liver failure is rare; symptoms are self-limited, and symptomatic treatment is the standard of care.

Evaluation

Given that the clinical presentation of HAV is nonspecific and the rate of HAV infection has decreased so dramatically, HAV infection should not be diagnosed on clinical features alone. Clinical suspicion is raised by an unvaccinated patient with recent exposure to HAV or participation in high-risk behaviors presenting with symptoms of fever, jaundice, nausea, vomiting, and joint pain. Evaluation of these patients should include liver functions tests, including serum total and unconjugated bilirubin, alkaline phosphatase, aspartate aminotransferase (AST) and alanine aminotransferase (ALT), prothrombin time/international normalized ratio, and albumin. Typical laboratory abnormalities include elevations in AST and ALT, total and direct bilirubin, and alkaline phosphatase levels. ALT is usually higher than AST, and elevations can be notable, usually ranging from 500 to 5000 IU/L. These laboratory abnormalities suggest the diagnosis of acute hepatitis; however, the diagnosis of *HAV* relies on positive serologic testing for HAV immunoglobulin M (IgM) antibodies, or proving a strong epidemiologic link to a laboratory-confirmed case of hepatitis A.[2] IgM anti-HAV becomes positive after 5 days of illness, but does not remain positive for long after the acute infection has resolved. It can also become positive shortly after receiving the HAV vaccine. Seventy-five percent of acute hepatitis cases are caused by either hepatitis A or hepatitis B, and appropriate laboratory evaluation should be undertaken in patients presenting with symptoms of acute viral hepatitis.[4]

Treatment

Treatment of HAV is very straightforward. Treatment is limited to supportive care as needed for nausea, vomiting, and other symptoms, as well as education to prevent further transmission, stressing proper hand hygiene. Patients should not return to school or work until fever and jaundice have resolved.[2,7]

Prevention

Prevention of HAV in the United States is largely accomplished through vaccination of all children at 1 year of age as well as adults deemed to be at high risk for HAV exposure which includes men who have sex with men, persons traveling to countries with high rates of hepatitis A, persons with risk for occupational exposure, persons with chronic liver disease, and household contacts of children recently adopted from hepatitis A endemic countries.[2] The HAV vaccine has greatly decreased the disease burden of hepatitis A in the United States. It is thought that the vaccine confers immunity for 25 years in adults and up to 20 years in children. There is no recommendation for booster doses at this time. Proper hand and surface hygiene at all times is also important prevention, especially during times of outbreak.[2,6]

Screening

Because hepatitis A does not develop into a chronic state, no screening is indicated. All persons desiring immunity can be vaccinated. There is no indication to check for natural immunity. If patients are unsure of vaccination history and desire immunity, they can be vaccinated, because there is no known serious harm from receiving a second vaccination.[2]

HEPATITIS B
Epidemiology

Routine vaccination of US children against the hepatitis B virus (HBV) began in 1991. In the last 20 years, HBV infection incidence in the United States has decreased 82%. However, unlike hepatitis A, acute HBV is more likely to be asymptomatic and can develop into a chronic infection. Even though the number of documented acute cases of HBV infection is similar to HAV, the estimated actual cases, clinical burden, and mortality from HBV are much higher. For example, in 2014, there were 2953 reported cases of acute HBV. However, acute HBV is only symptomatic 50% of the time; therefore, true acute cases are likely underreported, and it is estimated that there were approximately 19,200 acute cases in 2014.[8]

Chronic hepatitis B (CHB) is a more widespread problem and is estimated to affect between 850,000 and 2 million people in the United States alone. There were an estimated 53,800 new cases of CHB reported annually from 2004 to 2008, of which 95% were in immigrants from countries where hepatitis B is endemic.[9] CHB infection has large implications for long-term health.

Virus Description

HBV is a double-stranded, enveloped, DNA virus of the Hepadnaviridae family. It is the smallest DNA virus known, with the DNA in a partly double-stranded, circular pattern.[1] It replicates in hepatocytes and causes dysfunction of the liver.[1]

Transmission and Risk Factors

HBV is transmitted via the percutaneous or permucosal route. It is transmitted when the blood, semen, or vaginal fluids of an infected individual enter an uninfected person's body. Transmission can occur during sexual intercourse, through sharing of needles, when blood from an affected individual enters another person via an open wound or mucosal surface, and vertically from mother to child during childbirth. It is not spread through casual contact, but can be spread through close personal contact, especially if there are any cuts, wounds, or loss of normal skin barriers between both parties.[1]

Incubation

The incubation period for HBV is variable, ranging from 45 to 180 days, which can make it difficult to determine where and when transmission occurred.[1] The hepatitis B surface antigen (HBsAg) can be detected in blood as early as 30 to 60 days after exposure.[1]

Clinical Illness

Acute
HBV infection can cause an acute viral hepatitis with clinical manifestations similar to HAV infection. However, acute HBV infection is asymptomatic in up to 50% of patients.[8] Jaundice is infrequent in young children, appearing in less than 10% of acute cases. It is more common in adults and older children, appearing during acute infection about 50% of the time. Symptoms are similar to those of HAV and include fever, malaise, abdominal pain, nausea, vomiting, and flulike symptoms.[1,8]

The laboratory workup for suspected acute HBV is identical to HAV and will show similar alterations in liver transaminases. During acute illness, there is a marked elevation of ALT and AST, at times greater than 1000. Bilirubin can be normal, especially if the patient is not jaundiced. Liver transaminases should return to normal within 4 months following acute infection. As in HAV infection, once acute hepatitis is identified, testing for HAV and HBV antibodies should be performed, because clinically, the

2 infections look very similar. An acute HBV infection will show a positive HBsAg and positive IgM HBV core antibodies (IgM anti-HBc), as further described in later discussion.[1,10,11]

Treatment of acute HBV is similar to HAV treatment and consists of supportive care. Very few cases will develop into fulminant hepatic failure. Patients greater than the age of 60 are more likely to develop severe disease. The CDC reports that the fatality rate for acute HBV infection is 0.5% to 1%.[8]

Hepatitis B Virus Laboratory Values

An HBV panel of tests can be overwhelming; however the laboratory values are very informative and help delineate active versus previous infection, and acute versus chronic infection.

Hepatitis B surface antibody
The simplest antibody to understand is the hepatitis B surface antibody (anti-HBs). The anti-HBs is a protective antibody that will neutralize the virus.[1] When this value is positive, it indicates that the patient has immunity to HBV and is therefore no longer susceptible to acute infection nor chronically infected (**Table 1**). This value is checked when evaluating for past immunization or past infection. The anti-HBs is protective; therefore, there is no need to check other laboratory values, because the patient is neither acutely nor chronically infected and is protected from future infection. It cannot differentiate whether a person is immune through vaccination or from previous natural infection.

Hepatitis B core antibody
Hepatitis B core antibody (anti-HBc) indicates infection from the natural HBV. The HBV vaccination only contains HBsAg. It does not contain core components of the virus. Therefore, the anti-HBc is only positive in patients who have been exposed to naturally occurring HBV. It becomes positive following the incubation period, generally at the onset of symptoms, and remains positive for the life of the patient. Although this antibody indicates the patient has been exposed to HBV, it does not determine if the infection is acute, chronic, or cleared (**Table 2**). Only the presence of anti-HBs determines if the patient has cleared the infection. The concurrent presence of anti-HBc indicates the patient is immune from a natural infection, whereas its absence indicates the patient is immune from vaccination.[1]

Hepatitis B surface antigen
The laboratory test most essential to understanding a patient's hepatitis B status is the HBsAg. If this value is positive, the patient is currently infected with HBV, either acutely or chronically (**Table 3**). It also indicates that the patient is infectious. If the HBsAg is negative, the patient is not currently infected. It does not distinguish past infection, only current infection. HBsAg remains positive for an average of 4 weeks, but will be become negative by 15 weeks in all patients who have not developed chronic infection.[8] Because the HBsAg is a marker of current infection, and it is known that a patient will have a positive anti-HBc value if their body has been exposed to the HBV, then it is

	Susceptible to Infection	Immune, from Vaccination	Immune, past Infection	Chronic Infection	Acute Infection
Anti-HBs	Negative	Positive	Positive	Negative	Negative

Table 1
Interpretation of hepatitis B virus surface antibody result

Table 2					
Interpretation of hepatitis B virus core antibody result					
	Susceptible to Infection	Immune from Vaccination	Immune, past Infection	Chronic Infection	Acute Infection
Anti-HBc	Negative	Negative	Positive	Positive	*Positive*

known that a positive HBsAg will always be accompanied by a positive anti-HBc. Also, because the HBsAg is a marker of current infection, it is known that the anti-HBs value will be negative, because the anti-HBs is a protective antibody and a marker of immunity.

Hepatitis B core antibody IgM
After a positive HBsAg, the next step is to determine if the patient has an acute or chronic HBV infection. The IgM antibody to HBV core components (IgM anti-HBc) remains positive for about 6 months after infection with HBV. If this value is positive, it indicates that the patient is acutely infected with HBV via a temporal association; if negative, the patient is chronically infected, because they have a positive HBsAg and the absence of the IgM anti-HBc means they must have been infected for more than 6 months (**Table 4**). **Table 5** demonstrates how to interpret all results together.

Chronic
Although acute HBV is similar in clinical symptoms to acute HAV, the true risk and morbidity of HBV comes from its transformation into a chronic infection. The risk of progression to chronic HBV is largely dependent on the age at which the patient acquires the acute infection. The risk of progression to chronic is highest if the infection is acquired perinatally, with 90% of perinatal HBV infections becoming chronic.[1,10] Children between the ages of 1 and 5 at the time of infection have a 25% to 50% risk of chronic infection. After age 6 years, there is a 10% risk of progression to chronic infection.[1]

Chronic HBV infection is defined as having a positive HBsAg for more than 6 months, because all patients that will naturally clear the virus will do so within 15 weeks following infection.[8] Once the patient has developed chronic HBV infection, they are at a significantly increased risk of developing chronic liver disease, including cirrhosis and hepatocellular carcinoma. Twenty-five percent of patients who develop CHB during childhood, and 15% of those who develop CHB later in life, will die prematurely from hepatocellular carcinoma or cirrhosis.[8] In the United States alone, this accounts for approximately 1800 deaths per year.[8]

After identification of a CHB infection, patients require further evaluation of liver function, monitoring for cirrhosis, and consideration for possible treatment.[12] Persistent replication of the HBV leading to inflammation, cirrhosis, and hepatocellular carcinoma is the major factor in the morbidity and mortality of CHB. The goals of therapy are to reduce viral replication and damage to the liver. CHB has 5 phases, each with different

Table 3					
Interpretation of hepatitis B virus surface antigen result					
	Susceptible to Infection	Immune from Vaccination	Immune from past Infection	Chronically Infected	Acutely Infected
HBsAg	Negative	Negative	Negative	Positive	Positive

Table 4
Interpretation of hepatitis B virus chronic immunoglobulin M antibody result

	Susceptible to Infection	Immune from Vaccination	Immune from past Infection	Chronically Infected	Acutely Infected
IgM anti-HBc				Negative	*Positive*

implications for treatment. The hepatitis B e antigen (HBeAg) is a marker of high levels of viral replication, and patients will start to develop anti-HBe as they are clearing the virus. Liver cirrhosis is linked to the immune response to HBV, and elevated ALT levels correlate with a high immune response, not necessarily a high viral load.[9]

Phases of Chronic Hepatitis B

There are 5 phases of chronic HBV infection, all of which have different implications for treatment and management.[12] Patients will not necessarily progress through every stage in order during their chronic infection.

Phases

1. Immune tolerant phase: In this phase, patients will have high levels of HBV replication but no identifiable immune response. The HBeAg is positive, because this is a marker of high viral replication. The inflammation and damage to the liver are thought to be related to the immune response, so during this phase, there is little to no fibrosis or inflammation of the liver (**Table 6**).[12]
2. Immune clearance phase (HBeAg-positive CHB): Patients will have high levels of HBV DNA and are HBeAg positive, similar to the immune tolerant phase, but because of high immune activity, there is elevation of the ALT and fibrosis and inflammation of the liver.
3. Low viral replication phase: During this phase, patients have developed anti-HBe and are no longer HBeAg positive; there are low levels of HBV replication and limited inflammation. Patients will still have a positive HBsAg and have not cleared the virus yet.
4. Reactivation phase (HBeAg-negative CHB): Following the loss of HBeAg and the development of anti-HBe, patients may go into this stage and develop fibrosis and inflammation. This stage is characterized by fluctuating levels of ALT.
5. Resolution: During this stage, patients will have cleared the virus and will become HBsAg negative.

Treatment options

Treatment is usually started when ALT levels are elevated, so the 2 most common phases that are treated are the immune clearance phase (HBeAg-positive CHB) and

Table 5
Interpretation of the hepatitis B panel of tests

	Susceptible to Infection	Immune from Vaccination	Immune from past Infection	Chronically Infected	Acutely Infected
Anti- HBs	−	+	+	−	−
Anti-HBc	−	−	+	+	+
HBsAg	−	−	−	+	+
IgM anti-HBc	−	−	−	−	+

+, positive; −, negative.

Table 6
Laboratory results and the phases of chronic hepatitis B

Phase	HBsAg	HBeAg	HBV DNA	Anti-Hbe	ALT
Immune tolerant	+ >6 mo	+	↑↑	−	Normal or slightly elevated
Immune clearance phase (HBe-Ag-positive CHB)	+ >6 mo	+	↑↑	−	↑↑
Low viral replication	+ >6 mo	−	↓	+	Normal
Reactivation phase (HBeAg-negative CHB)	+ >6 mo	−	↑	+	↑↑
Resolution	−	−	Undetectable	+	Normal

↑↑, markedly elevated; ↑, mildly elevated; ↓, low.

the reactivation phase (HBeAg-negative CHB).[9] There are currently 7 medications indicated for treatment of CHB. There are 5 oral nucleotide reverse transcriptase inhibitors as well as pegylated interferon alfa-2a and interferon.

The preferred first-line agents at this time are entecavir, tenofovir, and pegylated interferon alfa-2a. The most common treatments at this time are 1 year of pegylated interferon alfa-2a or prolonged treatment with an oral nucleotide reverse transcriptase inhibitor.[9]

Screening

The US Preventive Services Task Force (USPSTF) recommends that all pregnant women in the United States be screened for HBV during their initial obstetrical laboratory work.[13] This screening allows physicians to identify women who are chronically infected with HBV and treat the infant at birth to prevent vertical transmission. All infants born to women who are infected with HBV are given hepatitis B immune globulin within 12 hours of birth and HBV vaccination at birth followed by appropriately timed second and third doses. This vaccination schedule decreases the risk of acute HBV infection in the infant to 4% to 10%, decreased from 90%.[9,14] Women who have high levels of HBV DNA during pregnancy have an increased risk of transmission to the fetus. Therefore, it is reasonable to start treatment in pregnant woman in the final trimester of pregnancy. Telbivudine and tenofovir are category B and can be considered for treatment.[9] Universal screening of all adults is not recommended, although it is a B recommendation by the USPSTF to screen adults who are at high risk for HBV exposure.[13]

Prevention

Immunization is recommended for all children beginning at birth in the United States. There are multiple other indications for vaccination, including all children less than 19 years who have not been vaccinated, men who have sex with men, and health care workers. There are multiple vaccination options, and all have different dosing schedules. Evidence suggests that the protection conferred by the vaccination lasts at least 20 years. There is no recommendation for a booster in immunocompetent individuals.[8]

Patients on hemodialysis should be screened yearly with an anti-HBs titer, as there are indications for booster vaccinations in hemodialysis patients. There is a recommendation to revaccinate hemodialysis patients when their titer of anti-HBs decreases to less than 10 mIU/mL. For other immunocompromised patients, there is a similar recommendation for yearly screening of anti-HBs titer and a consideration of a booster vaccination if their titers decrease to less than 10 mIU/mL.[8]

REFERENCES

1. Mahoney FJ. Update on diagnosis, management, and prevention of hepatitis B virus infection. Clin Microbiol Rev 1999;12(4):351–66.
2. Centers for Disease Control and Prevention. Hepatitis A FAQs for health professionals. Available at: http://www.cdc.gov/hepatitis/HAV/HAVfaq.htm. Accessed December 1, 2016.
3. Cuthbert JA. Hepatitis A: old and new. Clin Microbiol Rev 2001;14(1):38–58.
4. Nainan OV, Xia G, Vaughan G, et al. Diagnosis of hepatitis A infection: a molecular approach. Clin Microbiol Rev 2006;19(1):63–79.
5. Vogt T, Wise MF, Bell BP, et al. Declining hepatitis A mortality in the United States during the era of hepatitis A vaccination. J Infect Dis 2008;197(9):1282–8.
6. Fiore AE, Wasley A, Bell BP. Prevention of Hepatitis A through active or passive immunization: recommendations of the Advisory Committee on Immunization Practices (ACIP). MMWR Recomm Rep 2006;55(RR-7):1–23.
7. Jeong SH, Lee HS. Hepatitis A: clinical manifestations and management. Intervirology 2010;53(1):15–9.
8. Centers for Disease Control and Prevention. Hepatitis B FAQs for health professionals. Available at: https://www.cdc.gov/hepatitis/hbv/hbvfaq.htm. Accessed December 1, 2016.
9. Martin P, Lau DT, Nguyen MH, et al. A treatment algorithm for the management of chronic hepatitis B virus infection in the United States: 2015 update. Clin Gastroenterol Hepatol 2015;13:2071–87.
10. Gitlin N. Hepatitis B: diagnosis, prevention and treatment. Clin Chem 1997;43(8 Pt 2):1500–6.
11. Kim WR. Epidemiology of hepatitis B in the United States. Hepatology 2009;49(5 suppl):S28–34.
12. European Association for the Study of the Liver. EASL clinical practice guidelines: management of chronic hepatitis B virus infection. J Hepatol 2012;57:167–85.
13. United States Preventive Services Task Force. Hepatitis B virus infection: screening, 2014. Available at: https://www.uspreventiveservicestaskforce.org/Page/Document/UpdateSummaryFinal/hepatitis-b-virus-infection-screening-2014?ds=1&s=hepatitis B. Accessed March 10, 2017.
14. Wiseman E, Fraser MA, Holden S, et al. Perinatal transmission of hepatitis B virus: an Australian experience. Med J Aust 2009;190:489–92.

Hepatitis C: A New Era

Dee Ann Bragg, MD[a],*, Ashley Crowl, PharmD[b], Emily Manlove, MD[c]

KEYWORDS

- Hepatitis C • Hepatic fibrosis • HCV • Direct-acting antivirals

KEY POINTS

- Hepatitis C virus (HCV) is a common but underdiagnosed infection that affects at least 2 million Americans, about half of whom are unaware that they are infected.
- Given its often asymptomatic initial course, screening for HCV in those with risk factors is of utmost importance in the primary care setting.
- HCV causes many hepatic and extrahepatic complications, including cirrhosis, hepatocellular carcinoma, and death.
- With the advent of direct-acting antivirals, treatment of HCV is more successful than ever.

EPIDEMIOLOGY

The hepatitis C virus (HCV) is a small, single-stranded RNA virus in the Flaviviridae family with 6 genotypes and a propensity to cause chronic infection.[1] Approximately 2.7 to 7.1 million Americans have chronic hepatitis C.[2,3] It is estimated that 16,000 to 75,000 deaths yearly are attributed to HCV, and more Americans die from HCV than any other infectious cause (including HIV, tuberculosis, and pneumococcal disease).[4] Hepatitis C is also a costly disease, and costs are increasing. The number of admissions in the United States related to HCV tripled from the time period of 2004 to 2005 to 2010 to 2011.[5] Costs of US hospitalizations have also tripled in that same period, from $0.9 billion to $3.5 billion. The financial burden is shifting from private insurers to Medicare as the baby-boomer generation ages.

PATHOPHYSIOLOGY
Transmission

HCV is primarily transmitted through percutaneous blood exposure, and injection drug use accounts for at least 60% of cases in the United States.[6] The prevalence of HCV

Disclosure Statement: The authors have nothing to disclose.
[a] Via Christi Family Medicine Residency, University of Kansas School of Medicine (KUSM)-Wichita, 1121 South Clifton Street, Wichita, KS 67218, USA; [b] University of Kansas School of Pharmacy, 1121 South Clifton Street, Wichita, KS 67218, USA; [c] University of Kansas School of Medicine (KUSM)-Wichita, 1010 North Kansas Street, Wichita, KS 67214, USA
* Corresponding author.
E-mail address: DeeAnn.Bragg@ascension.org

among persons who inject drugs is approximately 50%.[7] Although sexual transmission is possible, it is generally inefficient except in cases of HIV coinfection or in men who have sex with men (MSM).[6]

Acute Phase

After contracting the virus, the incubation period lasts 2 to 26 weeks. The acute phase of infection lasts 1 to 3 weeks and is rarely symptomatic enough to be clinically evident. Although possible, hepatitis with acute liver failure is very rare in the acute setting.[8] At this time, however, HCV RNA is elevated and detectable, and serum transaminases are also elevated. Some individuals mount a robust immune response with T cells and thus clear the virus. Of patients infected, 20% to 50% will clear the virus and recover from the acute infection.[1] However, 50% to 80% are unable to clear the infection because the virus has several mechanisms to elude the immune system; these patients develop chronic hepatitis C.

Chronic Phase

The chronic phase of HCV infection is variable.[9] HCV directly impacts the liver by effectively creating an environment of low-grade hepatic inflammation. This inflammatory environment stimulates hepatic stellate cells to transform into myofibroblasts, thus leading to the production and accumulation of matrix proteins within the liver.[10] Some patients exhibit a mild progression of hepatitis, where inflammation is only seen in the portal tracts so that the liver architecture is maintained properly. Even in the mildest forms, hepatocyte apoptosis will still occur. Bridging necrosis and fibrosis between the portal tracts and hepatic veins is seen in advancing disease.

The result of ongoing hepatocyte destruction and fibrosis is cirrhosis. Given the largely asymptomatic initial course of acute and early chronic HCV and resulting delayed clinical diagnosis, it is difficult to determine the typical time frame for developing HCV-related cirrhosis. The overall risk appears to be about 15%, although cirrhosis can take up to 20 years after infection to become clinically apparent.[11,12] Once an HCV-infected patient becomes cirrhotic, the risk of developing liver failure, hepatocellular carcinoma (HCC), or liver-related death is about 3% for each outcome annually.[13] HCV is the underlying cause of one-half of liver disease cases in the United States.[9] Of patients with end-stage liver disease waiting for a liver transplant, 35% have HCV.[14]

DIAGNOSIS
Risk Assessment

Approximately half of those infected with HCV are unaware that they have the virus. Therefore, a major part of HCV diagnosis is the screening of asymptomatic but at-risk individuals. Risk factors include the following:

- Injection or intranasal drug use
- Unregulated tattoos
- Needle stick injuries
- Long-term hemodialysis
- HCV-infected mother
- Blood transfusion or organ transplant before 1992
- Incarceration
- Concomitant HIV infection

In addition, given exposures and behaviors within this particular birth cohort and a 5 times greater prevalence than other populations, all asymptomatic patients born between 1945 and 1965 should be offered one-time HCV screening. Testing should also be completed in patients with unexplained liver dysfunction or persistently elevated transaminase levels.[15]

Choice of Screening Test

There are traditionally 2 stages to diagnosing HCV infection: an initial antibody screen followed by a confirmatory virologic assay. Two-step testing is necessary because antibody tests are insensitive in the early stages of infection and lack the ability to differentiate acute disease from chronic or recovered states. In addition, false positive antibody results can occur in low-titer samples.[6]

The presence of circulating anti-HCV antibodies is detected using either enzyme immunoassay (EIA; or enzyme-linked immunosorbent assay) or chemiluminescence assay (CLIA). Clinically, these serum assays are ordered as a "Hepatitis C Antibody Test" or "Anti-HCV Antibody"; they are 97% to 98% sensitive and specific.[6] In low-resource settings, rapid diagnostic tests (RDTs) appear to increase diagnosis of high-risk individuals and should be considered for initial HCV antibody testing.[16] RDTs are available as either blood or oral fluid–based studies, have comparable sensitivity and specificity (83%–100% and 99%–100%, respectively), require little laboratory infra-structure, and are less costly than their EIA and CLIA counterparts.[17] Although sensitivity and specificity of antibody tests are high in the general population, immunocompro-mised patients (eg, those with HIV or on hemodialysis) may have an impaired antibody response and thus false negative results (specificity 65%–89%).[6,18] **Table 1** summarizes the best initial screening tests to order in a variety of clinical scenarios.

Approach to the Positive Antibody

In patients with positive antibody testing, a follow-up virologic study should be ordered to determine the presence or absence of current hepatitis C infection. The confirmatory study of choice is the HCV RNA test, which can be ordered as either a quantitative or a qualitative measure; both methods use nucleic acid testing (NAT) and are reliable mea-sures of viral replication. HCV RNA is detectable in serum 1 to 2 weeks after an initial infection. Although quantitative tests are more revealing in that they report a standard measure of international units per milliliter (also known as a "viral load"), the qualitative study has traditionally had the advantage of detecting the presence of circulating virus at lower levels than many of its quantitative counterparts.[19] However, it is currently rec-ommended that either measure of HCV RNA (whether qualitative or quantitative) must have a threshold of detection of 25 IU/mL or lower in order to be clinically useful.[15]

Although not currently available in every practice setting, the HCV core antigen test could be considered over HCV RNA testing in some clinical scenarios. Core antigen testing nears 100% specificity and is less labor intensive with a lower risk of laboratory contamination than NAT technology.[6] In very high-prevalence settings, it could also be used as a one-step diagnostic approach.[17] However, there is lacking evidence to recommend one-step core antigen testing over 2-step or HCV RNA testing in most situations. **Fig. 1** visually summarizes the stepwise process to diagnosing hepatitis C.

FIBROSIS STAGING
METAVIR System

Once HCV infection has been identified, it is important for prognostic and therapeutic purposes to evaluate the extent of fibrosis that has occurred in the liver. Clinically,

Table 1
Summary of screening recommendations for hepatitis C virus infection

Risk Factor	Preferred Initial Screening Test	Need for Ongoing Assessment/Screening?	Notes
Injection or intranasal drug use	HCV antibody	Yes, if risk behavior continues	Screen even if patient has only used once
Unregulated tattoo recipient	HCV antibody and HCV RNA	Yes, if ongoing risk/exposure	Tattoos received in state-regulated parlors should be safe
Incarceration	HCV antibody	No (once only unless other risk factors)	Risk includes current or past incarceration
Blood transfusion or organ transplant before 1992 or receipt of clotting factors before 1987	HCV antibody	No (once only)	Also test in those who were notified following a transfusion that the donor tested positive for HCV
US-born between 1945 and 1965	HCV antibody	No (once only), unless other ongoing risk factor	75% of those with the virus are in this birth cohort
Long-term hemodialysis (ever)	HCV antibody	No	HCV Ab not reliably detectable given immunocompromise
HIV infection	HCV antibody AND HCV RNA	Annually in HIV-positive MSM	HCV Ab not reliably detectable given immunocompromise
Children born to HCV-infected mothers	HCV RNA twice between 2 and 6 mo of age OR HCV Ab after 15 mo of age	No (see guidelines)	Per National Institutes of Health Consensus Guidelines

Adapted from AASLD/IDSA HCV Guidance Panel. Hepatitis C guidance: AASLD-IDSA recommendations for testing, managing, and treating adults infected with hepatitis C virus. Hepatology 2015;62(30):933–4; with permission.

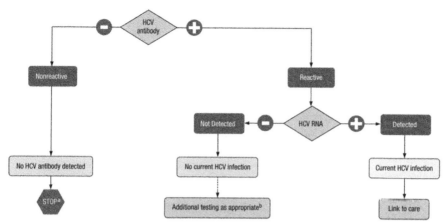

Fig. 1. Recommended testing sequence for identification of current HCV infection. [a] For persons who might have been exposed to HCV within the past 6 months, testing for HCV RNA or follow-up testing for HCV antibody is recommended. For persons who are immunocompromised, testing for HCV RNA can be considered. [b] To differentiate past, resolved HCV infection from biologic false positivity for HCV antibody, testing with another HCV antibody assay can be considered. Repeat HCV RNA testing if the person tested is suspected to have had HCV exposure within the past 6 months or has clinical evidence of HCV disease, or if there is concern regarding the handling or storage of the test specimen. (*From* Centers for Disease Control and Prevention (CDC). Testing for HCV infection: an update of guidance for clinicians and laboratorians. MMWR Morb Mortal Wkly Rep 2013;62:362–5; with permission.)

hepatic fibrosis can be staged using various scoring methods, the best studied of which is the METAVIR system. Using this system, a patient's fibrosis score ranges along a spectrum from F0 (no fibrosis) to F4 (cirrhosis). F1, F2, and F3 represent interval stages preceding cirrhosis but with progressively increasing bridging septum formation.[20] A METAVIR score is determined by 1 of 3 techniques, each with similar performance: liver biopsy, serum assay, or ultrasound-based testing.[21]

Liver Biopsy

Liver biopsy has been the historical gold standard of fibrosis assessment because it provides information regarding other predictive and prognostic processes, including inflammation, steatosis, and necrosis. However, biopsy is limited by its invasive risk, contraindications, and cost; additionally, it is fraught with potential sampling error in that a small specimen may not accurately represent the liver as a whole.[22] As other means of assessing fibrosis have become available and current treatments hold fewer risks and better outcomes, liver biopsies have become less standard in the management of hepatitis C.

Serum Testing for Fibrosis

There are several available serum tests for fibrosis, broadly classified as either direct or indirect. Indirect tests comprise simple serum measurements reflecting portal hypertension, liver dysfunction, or inflammation. They can be combined to produce diagnostic panels such as the aspartate aminotransferase (AST) to platelet ratio index (APRI), calculated as follows: (AST/upper limit of normal for sampling laboratory test)

× 100/platelet count. The higher the resulting number, the more likely the presence of significant fibrosis.

Direct tests measure markers of collagen synthesis or degradation, the most validated of which is hyaluronic acid. Several available tests combine direct and indirect markers, often also taking into account patient age and sex, and provide a resulting METAVIR score. Of these, the most widely validated and available in the United States is the FibroSURE test.[22] Although APRI and FibroSURE perform similarly, the former is less predictive because of the possibility of extrahepatic causes of thrombocytopenia or transaminitis, and the latter is significantly more costly.[23]

Imaging for Fibrosis

Imaging techniques for the measurement of fibrosis include ultrasound, computed tomography, and MRI-based methods. The most broadly used is transient elastography (TE; FibroScan), which uses an ultrasound transducer along with a vibrating device that releases low-frequency shearing waves; the speed of wave transmission is directly related to liver stiffness. Although this is a more accurate measure of cirrhosis than fibrosis, it can be used for either. Testing accuracy is further limited by several factors, including the presence of obesity, ascites, and acute hepatic inflammation. Magnetic resonance elastography is clinically superior to TE in that it visualizes the entirety of the liver with fewer patient-factor limitations, but is more cost-prohibitive and generally less available in many testing centers.[22]

CLINICAL MANIFESTATIONS
Hepatic Manifestations

Cirrhosis
Ongoing liver fibrosis leads to cirrhosis, which manifests clinically in a variety of ways, including but not limited to the following:

- Esophageal varices
- Hepatomegaly
- Ascites
- Gynecomastia
- Infertility and anovulation
- Spider angiomas
- Palmar erythema[24]

Cirrhosis is also reflected in several typical laboratory findings, including pancytopenia, transaminitis, increased bilirubin, and dilutional hyponatremia.

Hepatocellular carcinoma
HCC is the most common primary liver malignancy and the ninth leading cause of cancer-related death in the United States. Cirrhosis of any origin is a risk factor for its development. The cycle of cell death and regeneration seen in chronic hepatitis C can increase the risk of accumulated mutations in hepatocyte DNA, malignantly transform the cells, and increase the risk of HCC.[9] Alcohol consumption, diabetes mellitus, and obesity appear to confer additional risk. HCC develops almost exclusively in the cirrhotic liver, although up to 8% of cases occur in severe fibrosis.[25]

There are unfortunately no pathognomonic symptoms of HCC and, given the overlap with cirrhosis, any potential clinical manifestations are typically already present. These limiting factors often leads to late-stage diagnosis of HCC, at which point no available treatment can increase survival. If discovered at an early enough stage, radiation and chemotherapy are possible treatment options, but the only available curative treatments for HCC are surgical resection and orthotopic liver transplant.[25]

Extrahepatic Manifestations

Although primarily affecting the liver, HCV should be considered a systemic disease in that it leads to the development of immunologic, autoimmune, and viral phenomena throughout the body.[26] An estimated 40% to 74% of HCV patients will develop at least one extrahepatic manifestation throughout the course of their illness, leading to increased treatment cost and overall economic burden.[26,27]

Those conditions with the strongest HCV association include the following:

- Mixed cryoglobulinemia
- B-cell non-Hodgkin lymphoma[28]

Other manifestations include the following:

- Lichen planus
- Type 2 diabetes mellitus
- Membranoproliferative glomerulonephritis
- Porphyria cutanea tarda
- Rheumatoid-like arthritis
- Depression[27,28]

Successful treatment does appear to improve many systemic manifestations, and in addition, decreases mortality.[28]

TREATMENT
Goals of Treatment

The ultimate goal of HCV treatment is to eradicate the infection. Successful eradication is defined as having an undetectable viral load 12 weeks following treatment completion, also termed sustained virologic response (SVR). SVR confers a 97% to 100% chance of being HCV RNA negative long term and can therefore be considered a "cure."[29] Once SVR is achieved, patients will continue to have a detectable HCV antibody, but this does not imply immunity.

Secondary goals of HCV treatment include reducing clinical sequelae as well as decreasing future transmission risk and prevalence. Achieving SVR decreases the risk of developing chronic HCV, end-stage liver disease, HCC, and death. Therefore, treatment is especially important in cases of compensated cirrhosis, advanced fibrosis staging, severe extrahepatic HCV, and history of liver transplant.[15]

Nonpharmacologic therapy

Lifestyle changes are recommended to help reduce consequences of HCV[30]; this includes avoiding alcohol use in order to decrease disease progression. Patients should also eat a balanced diet and exercise regularly to obtain or maintain a normal weight, thus reducing the risk of concomitant nonalcoholic fatty liver disease or nonalcoholic steatohepatitis. Tobacco use can also contribute to disease progression, and a study comparing daily with occasional cannabis use in the setting of HCV infection showed higher rates of moderate to severe fibrosis in the daily users. Therefore, cessation of both tobacco and cannabis should be encouraged.[31] HCV patients should additionally be vaccinated against hepatitis A and B, and cirrhotic patients should receive pneumonia vaccination.[32] Last, patients should be educated on how to minimize HCV transmission by avoiding the following[33]:

- Sharing or reuse of needles, syringes, and other injectable devices
- Sharing personal items that may be infected (razor, toothbrush, nail-clippers)
- Acquiring tattoos or piercings from an unlicensed facility

Pharmacologic therapy

Interferon regimens After the discovery of HCV in 1989, interferon (IFN) was for several years the only HCV treatment regimen available and remained a staple of its management until 2012. It was originally used to treat hepatitis B before its use to treat HCV. Unfortunately, IFN was limited by poor efficacy with SVR rates of 15% to 20%.[34] In addition, IFN was associated with several intolerable side effects, such as neutropenia, myalgia, influenza-like symptoms, autoimmune disorders, depression, or other neuropsychiatric disturbances. These limiting clinical factors led to frequent discontinuation of IFN therapy by patients, which also contributed to poor SVR rates.

Ribavirin In the late 1990s, ribavirin was added to IFN regimens and improved SVR rates significantly to 38% to 56%.[34] Ribavirin is a nucleoside analogue, but the mechanism of its augmenting effects is not well known. This medication requires close therapeutic monitoring because it can cause hemolytic anemia. It can also worsen cardiac disease, leading to myocardial infarction. Ribavirin cannot be used in pregnant women because it is a pregnancy category X medication. When used in women of childbearing age, 2 forms of contraception are required during treatment and for 6 months after. Although use of ribavirin is diminishing, it is still used in combination with direct-acting antivirals (DAAs) in certain patients, such as those previously exposed to treatment or those with cirrhosis.[35]

Direct-acting antivirals In 2013, the first DAA was approved, drastically changing the landscape of HCV treatment. DAAs are now recommended for first-line management. They have improved SVR rates to 95% to 100% and have created the option of IFN-free regimens.[36] Although these medications are all broadly categorized as DAAs, they do have different mechanisms of action. The first 2 brought to market were protease inhibitors, boceprevir and telaprevir. Both still required use with IFN and ribavirin and had a limiting side-effect profile, which led to discontinuation of these medications in the US market when more tolerable agents were made available. The remaining DAAs affect HCV replication by targeting crucial viral proteins that inhibit the replication process. Specific types of available DAAs include HCV serine proteases, nonstructural protein inhibitors, nucleotide analogue inhibitors, nucleoside analogue inhibitors, and nonnucleoside inhibitors the remaining DAAs target crucial viral proteins and thus inhibit the HCV replication process.[34]

Each DAA is active against certain genotypes of the virus. The most common genotypes in the United States are 1, 2, and 3 and account for 97% of cases.[1] When selecting a DAA, patient genotype, cost, potential drug interactions, and side effects should be considered (**Table 2**). As DAAs are a new, innovative treatment of HCV, they have a high market value, ranging from $60,000 to 90,000 for one course of treatment.[34] However, DAAs have a more tolerable side-effect profile, fewer drug interactions, and an easier dosing schedule than IFN or ribavirin. These factors have allowed the management of HCV to occur in a primary care setting in some cases, as opposed to specialty environments only.

Table 2
Directing-acting antiviral medication chart

Medication, Brand (Generic)[a]	Genotypes Covered	Side Effects	Contraindications	Duration of Therapy, wk	SVR Rates, %	Other
Epclusa[37] (sofosbuvir/velpatasvir)	1, 2, 3, 4, 5, 6	Headache, fatigue	Coadministration with amiodarone	12	97–100	Used with ribavirin in decompensated cirrhosis
Zepatier[38] (elbasvir/grazoprevir)	1, 4	Headache, fatigue, and nausea	Moderate-severe hepatic impairment, use with OATP inhibitors/CYP3A inducers[b]/efavirenz	12–16	95–100	Used with ribavirin in treatment, experienced or NS5A polymorphisms
Daklinza[39] (daclatasvir)	1, 3	Headache, fatigue	CYP3A inducers[b]	12	82–100	Used with sofosbuvir; used with ribavirin in decompensated cirrhosis
Technivie[40] (ombitasvir/paritaprevir/ritonavir)	4	Asthenia, fatigue, nausea, insomnia	Moderate-severe hepatic impairment, CYP3A inducers,[b] sensitivity to ritonavir or ribavirin, ethinyl estradiol	12	91–100	Used with ribavirin
Viekira Pak[41] (ombitasvir/paritaprevir/ritonavir + dasabuvir)	1	Fatigue, nausea, pruritus, insomnia, asthenia	Severe hepatic impairment, CYP3A inducers,[b] CYP2C8 strong inducers and inhibitors, ethinylestradiol	12–24	95–100	Used with ribavirin in decompensated cirrhosis
Harvoni[42] (ledipasvir/sofosbuvir)	1, 4, 5, 6	Headache, fatigue, asthenia	Coadministration with amiodarone or P-gp inducers	12–24	93–98	Used with ribavirin in cirrhosis or treatment, experienced
Sovaldi[43] (sofosbuvir)	1, 2, 3, 4	Fatigue, headache	Coadministration with amiodarone	24	80–94	Used with ribavirin or IFN
Olysio[44] (simeprevir)	1	Headache, fatigue, nausea, photosensitivity/rash	Coadministration with amiodarone or P-gp inducers	12–24	90–96	Used with sofosbuvir or ribavirin/IFN

Abbreviations: OATP, Organic Anion Transporting Polypeptides; P-gp, P glycoprotein.
[a] Medications listed in order of approval to market (newest to oldest).
[b] Strong inducers of CYP3A include phenytoin, carbamazepine, rifampin, St. John's wort.

General Monitoring

It is imperative that providers maintain close patient follow-up when initiating HCV therapy in order to ensure both medication adherence and tolerance. Furthermore, several laboratory tests should be obtained during and after treatment, but specific monitoring will depend on which regimen is chosen.[15] After completing 4 weeks of treatment with a DAA alone, the following laboratory tests should be obtained:

- Complete blood count (CBC)
- Creatinine with estimated glomerular filtration rate
- Hepatic function panel
- HCV RNA quantitative testing (recheck at week 6 if detectable)

If the HCV RNA (viral load) level has increased by >1 log at week 6, the treatment regimen should be discontinued. HCV RNA should also be checked 12 weeks after completing treatment to evaluate for SVR. Additional laboratory tests or monitoring may be needed for each individual agent; please refer to specific medication package inserts for more details. Patients should also be assessed for any ongoing risk factors for HCV reinfection (intravenous or intranasal drug use), hepatic toxicity (alcohol abuse), and risk of hepatitis B virus reactivation (if patient had positive hepatitis B virus core antibody).

Following treatment, even with obtainment of SVR, those with severe fibrosis (META-VIR F3-F4) or clinical cirrhosis require ongoing surveillance for both HCC and esophageal varices. Ongoing surveillance is achieved with liver ultrasound every 6 months and routine endoscopy, respectively. Serum alpha-fetoprotein lacks sensitivity and specificity as a screening test and is not recommended for HCC surveillance.[45]

Finally, all patients who fail to achieve SVR should be monitored with CBC, comprehensive metabolic panel, and international normalized ratio every 6 to 12 months and should be considered for re-treatment as new options become available.

REFERENCES

1. Wilkins T, Akhtar M, Gititu E, et al. Diagnosis and management of hepatitis C. Am Fam Physician 2015;91(12):835–42.
2. Denniston MM, Jiles RB, Drobeniuc J, et al. Chronic hepatitis C virus infection in the United States, National Health and Nutrition Examination Survey 2003 to 2010. Ann Intern Med 2014;160(5):293–300.
3. Chak E, Talal AH, Sherman KE, et al. Hepatitis C virus infection in USA: an estimate of true prevalence. Liver Int 2011;31(8):1090–101.
4. Ly KN, Hughes EM, Jiles RB, et al. Rising mortality associated with hepatitis C virus in the United States, 2003-2013. Clin Infect Dis 2016;62(10):1287–8.
5. Xu F, Tong X, Leidner AJ. Hospitalizations and costs associated with hepatitis C and advanced liver disease continue to increase. Health Aff (Millwood) 2014; 33(10):1728–35.
6. Kesli R, Polat H, Terzi Y, et al. Comparison of a newly developed automated and quantitative hepatitis C virus (HCV) core antigen test with the HCV RNA assay for clinical usefulness in confirming anti-HCV results. J Clin Microbiol 2011;49(12):4089–93.
7. Armstrong GL, Wasley A, Simard EP, et al. The prevalence of hepatitis C virus infection in the United States, 1999 through 2002. Ann Intern Med 2006; 144(10):705–14.
8. Lauer GM, Walker BD. Hepatitis C virus infection. N Engl J Med 2001;345(1): 41–52.

9. Theise N. Liver and gallbladder. In: Kumar V, Abbas A, Aster J, editors. Pathologic basis of disease. 9th edition. Philadelphia: Saunders Elsevier; 2015. p. 821–81.

10. van der Meer AJ, Berenguer M. Reversion of disease manifestations after HCV eradication. J Hepatol 2016;65(1 Suppl):S95–s108.

11. Thein HH, Yi Q, Dore GJ, et al. Estimation of stage-specific fibrosis progression rates in chronic hepatitis C virus infection: a meta-analysis and meta-regression. Hepatology 2008;48(2):418–31.

12. Butt AA, Yan P, Lo Re V 3rd, et al. Liver fibrosis progression in hepatitis C virus infection after seroconversion. JAMA Intern Med 2015;175(2):178–85.

13. Singal AG, Volk ML, Jensen D, et al. A sustained viral response is associated with reduced liver-related morbidity and mortality in patients with hepatitis C virus. Clin Gastroenterol Hepatol 2010;8(3):280–8, 288.e1.

14. Wong RJ, Aguilar M, Cheung R, et al. Nonalcoholic steatohepatitis is the second leading etiology of liver disease among adults awaiting liver transplantation in the United States. Gastroenterology 2015;148(3):547–55.

15. AASLD/IDSA HCV Guidance Panel. Hepatitis C guidance: AASLD-IDSA recommendations for testing, managing, and treating adults infected with hepatitis C virus. Hepatology 2015;62(3):932–54.

16. Coats JT, Dillon JF. The effect of introducing point-of-care or dried blood spot analysis on the uptake of hepatitis C virus testing in high-risk populations: a systematic review of the literature. Int J Drug Pol 2015;26(11):1050–5.

17. Centers for Disease Control and Prevention (CDC). Testing for HCV infection: an update of guidance for clinicians and laboratorians. MMWR Morb Mortal Wkly Rep 2013;62(18):362–5.

18. Colin C, Lanoir D, Touzet S, et al. Sensitivity and specificity of third-generation hepatitis C virus antibody detection assays: an analysis of the literature. J viral Hepat 2001;8(2):87–95.

19. Pawlotsky JM. Use and interpretation of virological tests for hepatitis C. Hepatology 2002;36(5 Suppl 1):S65–73.

20. Saludes V, Gonzalez V, Planas R, et al. Tools for the diagnosis of hepatitis C virus infection and hepatic fibrosis staging. World J Gastroenterol 2014;20(13):3431–42.

21. Castera L, Vergniol J, Foucher J, et al. Prospective comparison of transient elastography, Fibrotest, APRI, and liver biopsy for the assessment of fibrosis in chronic hepatitis C. Gastroenterology 2005;128(2):343–50.

22. Almpanis Z, Demonakou M, Tiniakos D. Evaluation of liver fibrosis: "Something old, something new…". Ann Gastroenterol 2016;29(4):445–53.

23. Chou R, Wasson N. Blood tests to diagnose fibrosis or cirrhosis in patients with chronic hepatitis C virus infection. Ann Intern Med 2013;159(5):372.

24. Fukui H, Saito H, Ueno Y, et al. Evidence-based clinical practice guidelines for liver cirrhosis 2015. J Gastroenterol 2016;51(7):629–50.

25. Balogh J, Victor D 3rd, Asham EH, et al. Hepatocellular carcinoma: a review. J Hepatocell Carcinoma 2016;3:41–53.

26. Gill K, Ghazinian H, Manch R, et al. Hepatitis C virus as a systemic disease: reaching beyond the liver. Hepatol Int 2016;10(3):415–23.

27. Younossi Z, Park H, Henry L, et al. Extrahepatic manifestations of hepatitis C: a meta-analysis of prevalence, quality of life, and economic burden. Gastroenterology 2016;150(7):1599–608.

28. Tang L, Marcell L, Kottilil S. Systemic manifestations of hepatitis C infection. Infect Agent Cancer 2016;11:29.

29. Simmons B, Saleem J, Hill A, et al. Risk of late relapse or reinfection with hepatitis C virus after achieving a sustained virological response: a systematic review and meta-analysis. Clin Infect Dis 2016;62(6):683–94.

30. Nobili V, Carter-Kent C, Feldstein AE. The role of lifestyle changes in the management of chronic liver disease. BMC Med 2011;9:70.

31. Ishida JH, Peters MG, Jin C, et al. Influence of cannabis use on severity of hepatitis C disease. Clin Gastroenterol Hepatol 2008;6(1):69–75.

32. Rubin LG, Levin MJ, Ljungman P, et al. 2013 IDSA clinical practice guideline for vaccination of the immunocompromised host. Clin Infect Dis 2014;58(3):309–18.

33. Alter MJ. Prevention of spread of hepatitis C. Hepatology 2002;36(5 Suppl 1): S93–8.

34. Heim MH. 25 years of interferon-based treatment of chronic hepatitis C: an epoch coming to an end. Nat Rev Immunol 2013;13(7):535–42.

35. Trepo C. A brief history of hepatitis milestones. Liver Int 2014;34(Suppl 1):29–37.

36. Lawitz E, Poordad FF, Pang PS, et al. Sofosbuvir and ledipasvir fixed-dose combination with and without ribavirin in treatment-naive and previously treated patients with genotype 1 hepatitis C virus infection (LONESTAR): an open-label, randomised, phase 2 trial. Lancet 2014;383(9916):515–23.

37. Epclusa® [package insert]. Foster City, CA: Gilead Sciences I; 2016.

38. Zepatier™ [package insert]. Kenilworth, NJ: Merck & Co I; 2016.

39. Daklinza™ [package insert]. NY: Bristol-Myers Squibb Company NY; 2015.

40. Technivie™ [package insert]. North Chicago, IL: AbbVie I; 2015.

41. Viekira Pak® [package insert]. North Chicago, IL: AbbVie I; 2014.

42. Harvoni® [package insert]. Foster City, CA: Gilead Sciences I; 2014.

43. Sovaldi® [package insert]. Foster City, CA: Gilead Sciences I; 2013.

44. Olysio® [package insert]. Titusville, NJ: Janssen Products L; 2013.

45. Bruix J, Sherman M. Management of hepatocellular carcinoma: an update. Hepatology 2011;53(3):1020–2.

Diverticular Disease of the Gastrointestinal Tract

 CrossMark

KEYWORDS

- Diverticular disease • Gastrointestinal tract • Esophagus • Stomach
- Small Intestine • Colon • Diverticular Bleeding • Diverticulosis

KEY POINTS

- Almost all gastrointestinal tract diverticula require no intervention if they are asymptomatic.
- There is no clear diagnostic modality of choice for diagnosis and surveillance of diverticulum.
- Medical treatment should be attempted before surgical intervention because significant morbidity is associated with resection.

ANATOMY AND CLASSIFICATION

Diverticula develop throughout the gastrointestinal tract because of a myriad of factors. The most common factors include abnormal pressure gradients, dysfunctional peristalsis, and defects of the bowel wall. In general, the gastrointestinal tract consists of the submucosal, mucosal, and muscular layers. A diverticulum is a pouch structure projecting outward from the canal and may contain one or more of these layers. In general, there are 2 broad categories of diverticula: true and false. A false diverticulum is a protrusion of the submucosa and mucosa through a defect in the muscular wall of the gastrointestinal tract. A true diverticulum is a protrusion of all layers of the gastrointestinal tract wall. This classification does not seem to impact decisions on treatment. Treatment is more directed by size, location, and symptoms of the diverticula.

ESOPHAGUS
Upper Esophagus

Zenker diverticulum is a false diverticulum that develops in the upper posterior esophagus. For unclear reasons, a Zenker diverticulum is more common in men and typically presents after the age of 60. It affects only 2 per 100,000 patients per year. Most upper esophageal diverticula are asymptomatic. Over time, patients may begin to experience symptoms of dysphagia, aspiration, and regurgitation of undigested food.

The author has nothing to disclose.
Department of Community and Family Medicine, University of Kansas School of Medicine, WesleyCare Family Medicine Center, 850 North Hillside Road, Wichita, KS 67214, USA
E-mail address: Aaron.Sinclair@wesleymc.com

Prim Care Clin Office Pract 44 (2017) 643–654
http://dx.doi.org/10.1016/j.pop.2017.07.007
0095-4543/17/© 2017 Elsevier Inc. All rights reserved.

A Zenker diverticulum develops in an area known as Killian triangle. The area is located between the inferior pharyngeal constrictors and the cricopharyngeal muscles. There appears to be an age-related descent of the larynx, which results in the inferior constrictor pharyngeal musculature taking an oblique course. This oblique course results in a weak spot and the subsequent potential for development of a false diverticulum. The exact cause is unclear, but proposed mechanisms suggest a combination of a dysfunction in coordinated swallowing-muscle movement and an increased intraluminal pressure in the esophagus. There may also be a component of long-term upper esophageal sphincter irritation from gastroesophageal reflux disease with Zenker diverticulum development.[1]

Diagnosis can be made endoscopically or radiologically. The preferred method is with barium swallow imaging, although small diverticulum may be difficult to identify (**Fig. 1**). Although endoscopic direct visualization is possible, caution should be exercised because of the risk of perforation with the blind insertion into the upper esophagus that occurs during endoscopy. Small asymptomatic diverticulum should be monitored, and regardless of symptoms, any Zenker diverticulum greater than 2 cm in size should be surgically evaluated and considered for repair. Methods for closure include endoscopic management or traditional surgical resection. Most advocate for endoscopic management because it is less invasive and has a lower complication rate and mortality.[2] There is a higher risk of recurrence with endoscopic repair versus surgical resection. More than 90% of patients will demonstrate symptom improvement; recurrence rates can be as high as 35%.[3]

Middle Esophagus

Traction diverticula are diverticula that form in the middle of the esophagus. These rare, true diverticula were named because of their proposed mechanism of formation. Their size tends to stay small, usually less than 2 cm. One possible mechanism is a precedent pulmonary infection (tuberculosis or histoplasmosis) that results in mediastinal lymph node formation. As the lymph nodes regress in size, fibrosis and scarring cause a traction point in the middle esophagus. This traction point serves as the initiation and is coupled with age-related changes from the dysfunction of coordinated swallowing-muscle movement and intraluminal pressure in the esophagus, which results in the formation of a diverticulum. It is unclear exactly how traction diverticulum

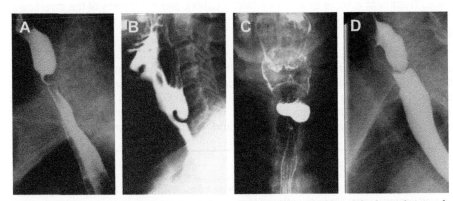

Fig. 1. Esophagram depicting (*A*) lateral view of a cricopharyngeal bar, (*B*) a lateral view of a small Zenker diverticulum, (*C*) its associated anterior-posterior view, and (*D*) a lateral view of a large Zenker diverticulum. (*From* Prisman E, Genden EM. Zenker diverticulum. Otolaryngol Clin North Am 2013;46(6):1101–11; with permission.)

develop and the importance of each component in the progression of the development of the diverticulum.[4]

Diagnosis can be made with endoscopy, barium swallow study, or computed tomography (CT). Treatment is rarely needed unless symptoms develop, and symptoms are largely related to the size of the diverticulum.

Lower Esophagus

An epiphrenic diverticulum is a false diverticulum in the lower third of the esophagus. These rare diverticula arise in only 0.015% of the population.[5] The formation of epiphrenic diverticula starts with mucosal injury from gastroesophageal reflux and continues with age-related muscle dysmotility. Because of its location, typically within 10 cm of the lower esophageal sphincter, symptoms may develop, including dysphagia, spasmodic chest pain, and heartburn.

Diagnosis can be made with endoscopy, barium swallow study, or CT. Epiphrenic diverticula that are small (<5 cm) and asymptomatic and can be monitored clinically or endoscopically for interval progression. As diverticular size increases, symptoms are likely to progress and potentially cause obstruction. Treatment plans for symptomatic epiphrenic diverticula require additional diagnostic testing, including 24-hour pH probe or esophageal manometry. This additional information on degrees of reflux may aid in the decision of open or laparoscopic diverticulum resection with possible fundoplication.[6]

STOMACH

Gastric diverticula may present anatomically in different locations of the stomach. True diverticula are located throughout the stomach, with false diverticula developing in the antrum region. The prevalence of gastric diverticula is approximately 0.04%. There does not appear to be a clear pathophysiologic mechanism for gastric diverticula formation. However, they appear to stay small in size (1–3 cm) and do not cause symptoms. Symptoms when they do occur include epigastric pain, dyspepsia, and emesis. Infrequently, ulcerations, perforations, or bleeding can occur.[7]

Diagnosis can be made with endoscopy, barium swallow study, or CT. Management should start with proton pump inhibitors if symptoms are present. If symptoms worsen or the diverticulum enlarges, then a gastrectomy may become necessary.[8]

SMALL INTESTINE

Duodenal diverticula are relatively common and seen in up to 22% of the population. Duodenal diverticula may be either true or false. The most common location is the second part of the duodenum (62%), followed by the third part of the duodenum (30%), and finally the fourth part of the duodenum (8%).[9] Duodenal diverticula are predominately false diverticula that develop because of a combination of intraluminal pressure and a weakness of the muscular wall. Although common, duodenal diverticula are largely asymptomatic and discovered incidentally. When symptoms develop, they can be significant because of proximity to adjacent structures and the size of the diverticulum. Symptoms may include obstruction, infection, jaundice, pain, perforation, or bleeding.

Diagnosis can be made with endoscopy, barium swallow study, or CT (**Fig. 2**). The CT scan gives additional information of the surrounding tissues and is often regarded as the test of choice for evaluation of the duodenal diverticulum. Evaluation of symptomatic diverticula includes either endoscopic intervention or surgical resection.[10] Surgical resection should not be performed unless significant symptoms are present because of a high risk of fistula formation and associated mortality of up to 30%.[9]

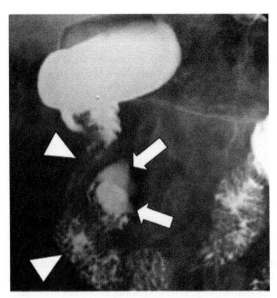

Fig. 2. Upper gastrointestinal series: duodenal diverticulum (*arrows*) arising on the internal border of D2 (*arrowheads*). (*From* Oukachbi N, Brouzes S. Management of complicated duodenal diverticula. J Visc Surg 2013;150(3):173–9; with permission.)

Jejunal and ileal diverticula appear throughout the remainder of the small intestine. The prevalence is 1% to 2% of the population. These false diverticula develop in areas of vasculature penetration of the muscular wall on the mesenteric side of the bowel wall. Jejunal and ileal diverticula are usually noted incidentally because of the largely asymptomatic nature of these diverticula. However, when symptoms develop, bleeding, diarrhea, obstruction, or infection may be present.[11]

Diagnosis can be made with small bowel barium contrast follow-through study, capsule endoscopy, and less commonly, CT scans with intravenous and oral contrast. Bacterial overgrowth symptoms may respond to antibiotic treatments and intestinal promotility drug treatment. Asymptomatic jejunal and ileal diverticula should not be resected. Surgical intervention with small bowel resection is reserved for persistently symptomatic ileal and jejunal diverticula.

MECKEL DIVERTICULUM

A Meckel diverticulum is the most common congenital anomaly affecting up to 4% of the general population. It is caused by an incomplete closure of the vitelline duct that typically recedes and involutes by the ninth gestational week of age. A Meckel's diverticulum is a true diverticulum because of its formation with all layers of the gastrointestinal tract. Most commonly remembered by the rule of 2's, Meckel diverticulum has several common characteristics (**Box 1**).[12]

The classic presentation is bloody mucoid stools, abdominal pain, and vomiting in a young child under the age of 6. Intussusception is a common cause of this presentation because of a remnant fibrous attachment to the umbilicus. This attachment allows the proximal bowel to involute onto the distal bowel. Ectopic mucosa located in the Meckel diverticulum may lead to other symptoms. Gastrointestinal bleeding or pain from ulcerations has been attributed to acid secretion by ectopic gastric mucosa. Although other tissues have been identified (duodenal and pancreatic), they tend to be rare and primarily asymptomatic.

Box 1
Meckel diverticulum characteristics

2% of the population

2% will become symptomatic

2 cm in length

2 inches in diameter

2 years of age or prior is the most common age of presentation

2 feet from the ileocecal valve

2:1 male-to-female ratio

2 types of ectopic tissues are most commonly identified if any

---

Diagnosis of a Meckel diverticulum requires attention to the differential diagnosis and a degree of suspicion. In children, signs of obstruction suggestive of intussusception can be best diagnosed with ultrasonography. However, local expertise may limit the usage of this modality, in which case CT scans may be used but may contain vague, broad findings that are suggestive, but not diagnostic, of a Meckel diverticulum.[13] Radiographic studies lack the necessary sensitivity and specificity to aid in the diagnosis of a Meckel diverticulum. Diagnosis in the adult patient requires a high index of suspicion. Because 23% to 50% of all Meckel diverticulum may have ectopic gastric mucosa, a technetium 99m (Tc^{99m}) scan to identify ectopic gastric mucosa may aid in the diagnosis[14] (**Fig. 3**). The sensitivity of the Meckel scan for the pediatric population is 85% to 97% but is much lower in the adult population at 62%.[15,16]

Table 1
Diverticula of the gastrointestinal tract

Location	Common Name	Type	Diagnosis	Treatment	Intervention Indication
Esophagus	Zenker	False	E, CT, S	Endoscopic or surgical resection	Symptomatic or >2 cm size
	Traction	True	E, CT, S	Surgical resection	Symptomatic
	Epiphrenic	False	E, CT, S	Laparoscopic surgical resection	Symptomatic or >5 cm size
Gastric	Gastric	Both	E, CT, S	Gastrectomy	Symptomatic, after failed proton pump inhibitors
Duodenum	Duodenal	Both	E, CT, S	Surgical resection	Significant symptoms
Jejunal	Jejunal	False	CT, S, P	Surgical resection	Significant symptoms; after failed promotility and antibiotics
Ileum	Ileal	False	CT, S, P	Surgical resection	Significant symptoms; after failed promotility and antibiotics
	Meckel	True	CT, M	Surgical resection	All symptomatic, asymptomatic with special inclusion criteria
Colon	Diverticulosis	False	E, CT, U	Rare	Only with severe complications

Abbreviations: E, endoscopy; M, Meckel scan; P, pill endoscopy; S, swallow study; U, ultrasound.

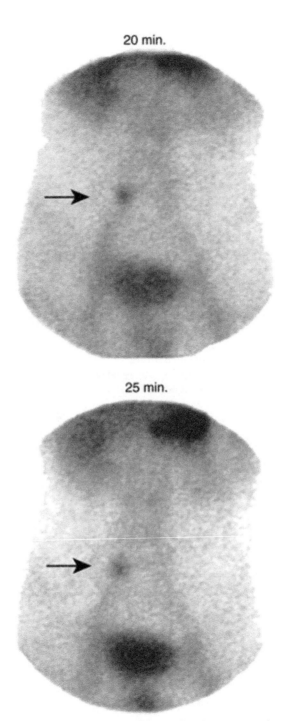

Fig. 3. Meckel scan demonstrating accumulation of technetium in the stomach superior bladder (inferior) and in the acid-secreting mucosa of a Meckel diverticulum. ->, indicates the duodenal diverticulum. (*From* Kliegman RM, Stanton BF, St Geme JW, et al. editors. Nelson textbook of pediatrics. Philadelphia: Elsevier; 2016. p. 1804–5.e1; with permission.)

All symptomatic Meckel diverticula should be surgically removed. Up to 90% of pediatric intussusceptions secondary to a Meckel diverticulum may be reduced during diagnostic ultrasonography. Debate continues with regard to the asymptomatic, incidentally noted Meckel diverticulum. Removal of asymptomatic diverticulum has been associated with a 5-fold increase in complications, such as postoperative bowel obstruction and infection. Therefore, many experts advocate no treatment or interventions.[17] Some experts will advocate for selective surgical resection in asymptomatic, incidentally noted Meckel diverticulum patients. Those asymptomatic, incidentally noted Meckel's diverticulum patients include healthy young children or healthy adults less than 50 years of age with any of the following: palpable abnormality suggestive of heterotropic tissue, size longer than 2 cm, or broad base wider than 2 cm.[18]

COLON

Diverticulosis is a common nomenclature for diverticula of the colon, which is the most common place that diverticula can occur in the gastrointestinal tract. A diverticulum in the colon is of the false type. The incidence of diverticulosis is 5% at age 40 and increases substantially over time to 60% at age 80. The most prominent location of the colon for diverticula is in the sigmoid region. A few risk factors have been noted for the development and propagation of diverticular disease: smoking, lack of physical activity, and obesity.[19]

The proposed mechanism of diverticular formation in the colon places an emphasis on intraluminal pressure buildup. The pressure across the colonic wall increases as the radius of the wall decreases. The sigmoid region of the colon is the smallest diameter and thus becomes the most likely location for diverticula to form. Early in life the pressure of the colon appears to be consistent throughout all segments of the bowel wall. However, as diverticular disease develops, this equal pressure is disrupted and pressure gradients develop. With increased pressure, the integrity of collagen and elastin (the structural framework of the colon) in the wall muscle changes. Next, the circular muscles thicken, colonic segments shorten, and finally, the lumen narrows. This entire process leads to the gradual increases in the severity and number of diverticula.[20]

The bulk of treatment efforts have focused on increasing the bulk of stool in the colon to help decrease the amount of pressure in the colon. Dietary fiber has been the predominant bulking agent studied. However, results have been inconclusive, and no consensus has been reached as to their benefit (**Table 1**).[21,22]

COLONIC DIVERTICULAR BLEEDING

Up to 15% of all patients with diverticulosis will experience a complication of bleeding diverticula in their lifetime. Diverticular bleeding is the cause of up to 50% of all hematochezia.[23] After one episode of diverticular bleeding, the recurrence rate of bleeding is estimated at 38%. The bleeding can vary from quite brisk to an intermittent dark, melenotic stool. The bleeding typically lacks accompanying symptoms, but may have associated nausea, bloating, and cramping.[24]

The cause of bleeding diverticula seems to be associated with the pathophysiology. Diverticula tend to develop where small arterioles penetrate the circular muscle of the colon. As the diverticulum enlarges, the stretching lumen drags the arteriole along the dome of the diverticula. This vessel is susceptible to damage and subsequent bleeding. Up to 50% of all diverticular bleeding originates from the right colon; this is suspected to be due to the thinner lumen noted in this region.

Endoscopy is most effective in diagnosing colonic diverticular bleeding. Up to 80% of all diverticular bleeding can be identified on direct endoscopic visualization.[25] Most bleeding diverticula can be stopped during endoscopy with hemostasis clips or subcutaneous epinephrine infusion. Many experts, because of its efficacy in identification and treatment, advocate for endoscopy to be done as soon as possible and preferably within 24 hours of admission. Nevertheless, some patients may not be hemodynamically stable to undergo urgent or emergent endoscopy upon presentation. In addition, although blood is a cathartic, if the bleeding seems to be slowing, some physicians advocate for a bowel preparation before endoscopy to increase the chances of identifying the source of bleeding. Hemodynamically unstable patients have a higher risk of adverse outcomes during endoscopic procedures or from the bowel preparation and sedation. Therefore, adequate fluid resuscitation, conservative blood transfusions, serial laboratory studies, and frequent patient assessments are necessary until endoscopy is deemed safe.

For some patients, endoscopy is not an option or does not isolate the source of bleeding. Patients with brisk or intermittent bleeding episodes may benefit from radiologic diagnosis. Radionuclide imaging requires that bleeding be active (minimum 0.05–0.1 mL/min) to accurately isolate the location of the diverticular source. Radionuclide imaging may use Tc^{99m} sulfur colloid autologous red blood cells because of its shorter half-life for active bleeding. However, ^{99m}Tc pertechnetate-labeled autologous red blood cells have a longer half-life and may be more beneficial in intermittent bleeding diverticula. Radionuclide imaging has a positive likelihood ratio of 51% in lower gastrointestinal bleeding.[26] Some experts advocate that radionuclide imaging be used as an ancillary test for directed angiography or possibly surgery. Angiography can be used in bleeding that is at least 0.5 mL/min with accuracy ranging from 40% to 78%. Another benefit of angiography is that catheter-directed embolization or vasopressin infusion can be used upon diagnostic localization of the diverticular bleeding to accomplish hemostasis. Unfortunately, angiography carries an increased risk of bowel infarction and contrast-induced nephrotoxicity.[27]

DIVERTICULITIS

Infection of colonic diverticula occurs in about 4% of all patients with diverticulosis.[28] Infection and inflammation of segmental portions of the colon affected by diverticula can range in severity from mild to severe.

The proposed mechanism of uncomplicated diverticulitis may start with a blocked diverticulum or trauma-associated mucosal injury. Either mechanism coupled with a component of deranged colonic bacterial flora leads to initial inflammation and infection. Expansion of the diverticula and surrounding tissue from inflammation and infection may result in compromised blood flow or microperforation. These microperforations may coalesce into localized abscess formation.

Complicated diverticulitis is classified when abscess formation extends beyond the colon into adjacent organs. This extension may present as fistulas, macroperforations, obstructions, or enlarging abscesses. This progression occurs in up to 25% of all cases of diverticulitis.

The age at presentation is typically in the sixth decade of life. The clinical presentation usually begins with mild abdominal pain with subsequent localization over the segment of colon affected, usually the sigmoid. Fever, nausea, and a change in bowel habits are also common features. If presentation to medical care is delayed, evidence of sepsis, peritoneal signs, or hemodynamic changes may be present.

The diagnosis is often made with the classical presentation of history, physical examination, radiographic imaging, and laboratory evaluation. Those patients with a past medical history of diverticulitis and presenting early in the disease process may be treated without laboratory or radiographic imaging as an outpatient with oral medications. Laboratory findings may include an elevated white blood cell count and inflammatory markers (C-reactive protein or erythrocyte sedimentation rate). If clinical presentation suggests sepsis, then blood cultures and lactic acid levels should be drawn at presentation. Radiographic imaging may initially include abdominal radiographs. However, findings are nonspecific and may include ileus, bowel perforation, or obstruction. Ultrasonography has sensitivities and specificities of 92% and 90% for the detection of diverticulitis. With sensitivities and specificities of 94% and 99%, CT appears to be the test of choice (**Fig. 4**). This is especially true as an alternative diagnosis was more likely to be identified with CT than with ultrasonography (50%–100% vs 33%–78%).[29]

The true benefit of antibiotics was questioned recently when a study showed no added benefit of antibiotics in uncomplicated diverticulitis. However, many experts argue that further studies are needed to confirm those findings and still agree that the mainstay of treatment of diverticulitis of any severity is antibiotic therapy (**Table 2**). Outpatient therapy is the preferred method if diverticulitis is diagnosed early. Inpatient therapy is recommended if complicated diverticulitis is diagnosed with radiographic studies or the patient has comorbid conditions, immunosuppression, high-grade fevers, leukocytosis, or is elderly. Diverticulitis is most commonly caused by gram-negative and anaerobic bacteria, and **Table 2** shows common antibiotic treatment options.[30] Patients should clinically improve within 48 hours of initiation of antibiotics and bowel rest. If improvement is not noted, reevaluation of the differential diagnosis or the severity of the diverticulitis should be completed. Part of that reevaluation could include repeat imaging, advanced imaging, or consideration for endoscopic evaluation. A focus of the differential diagnosis in nonimprovers should include inflammatory bowel disease or colon cancer. As the patient begins to improve, stool softeners and a high-fiber diet should be initiated to help lower intraluminal pressure and continued indefinitely.

Complicated diverticulitis associated with abscess formation should be managed in consultation with a surgeon for surgical evaluation or an interventional radiologist for percutaneous drainage. Depending on location, abscesses can be drained transanally

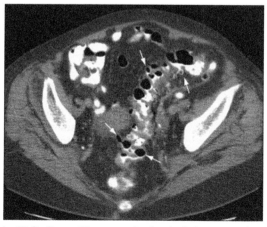

Fig. 4. Diverticulosis: CT findings. CT scan at the level of the sigmoid colon shows multiple air- and contrast-filled diverticula (*arrows*). (*From* Gore RM, Levine MS. Diverticulosis. In: High-yield imaging: gastrointestinal. Philadelphia: Elsevier; 2010. p. 382–4; with permission.)

Table 2
Antibiotic therapy for diverticulitis

Medication	Dosage
Uncomplicated diverticulitis (outpatient management)	
Amoxicillin-clavulanate	875 mg PO every 12 h
Ciprofloxacin and metronidazole	500 mg PO every 12 h 500 mg PO every 8 h
Levofloxacin and metronidazole	500 mg PO every 24 h 500 mg IV every 8 h
Moxifloxacin	400 mg PO every 24 h
	Duration: 10–14 d
Complicated diverticulitis (inpatient management)	
Ceftriaxone and metronidazole	1 g IV every 24 h 500 mg IV every 8 h
Imipenem-cilastatin	500 mg IV every 6 h
Levofloxacin and metronidazole	500 mg IV every 24 h 500 mg IV every 8 h
Piperacillin-tazobactam	3.375 g IV every 6 h
Ticarcillin-cilastin	3.1 g IV every 4 h
	Total PO and IV treatment 10–14 d

Clindamycin may be substituted in metronidazole intolerance/allergy.
Abbreviations: IV, intravenous; PO, by mouth.
Data from Jacobs DO. Clinical practice. Diverticulitis. N Engl J Med 2007;357:2057–66.

through drainage tube placement or aspiration completed under CT or ultrasound guidance. A general recommendation exists for consideration of drainage (preferably with interventional radiology) for any abscess measuring greater than 3 to 4 cm.[31]

Standard practice for many years has been to recommend endoscopic evaluation of the colon after the resolution of the first case of diverticulitis. Significant overlaps of CT scan features exist between colon cancer and diverticulitis.[32] Therefore, an underlying colon cancer cannot always be excluded with the initial diagnosis of diverticulitis. Colonoscopy is therefore typically recommended to rule out colon cancer 3 to 6 weeks after resolution of the diverticulitis. If a screening colonoscopy has been completed recently, then a repeat may not be necessary.

Extensive research is being conducted with regard to prevention of recurrent diverticulitis. Fiber may be used as a beneficial supplement to prevent recurrence of complications from underlying diverticulum. For years, popcorn seeds and nuts have been blamed as a cause of diverticulitis. Studies have shown no causal relationship, and thus, these foods are safe to consume for patients with diverticulosis or diverticulitis. Probiotics have not been shown to prevent recurrence.[25] However, mesalamine and rifaximin, in combination or alone, may help prevent recurrent episodes of diverticulitis.[33]

If recurrent diverticulitis is not prevented, consideration for segmental colectomy can be considered. Debate still exists as to the ideal patient or optimal timing for greatest benefit. However, if a patient is older than 50 and has had at least 4 recurrences of diverticulitis, surgical consultation with discussion of benefits and risks of surgery, compared with the risks of recurrent diverticulitis, should be offered. There is insufficient evidence to make a recommendation in younger patients or those with fewer recurrences of diverticulitis.[25]

REFERENCES

1. Prisman E, Genden EM. Zenker diverticulum. Otolaryngol Clin North Am 2013;46: 1101–11.
2. Verdonck J, Morton RP. Systematic review on treatment of Zenker's diverticulum. Eur Arch Otorhinolaryngol 2015;272:3095–107.
3. Johnson CM, Postma GN. Zenker diverticulum – which surgical approach is superior? JAMA Otolaryngol Head Neck Surg 2016;142:401–2.
4. do Nascimento FA, Lemme EM, Costa MM. Esophageal diverticula: pathogenesis, clinical aspects, and natural history. Dysphagia 2006;21:198–205.
5. Maish MS. Esophagus. In: Townsend CM Jr, Beauchamp D, editors. Townsend: Sabiston textbook of surgery. 19th edition. Philadelphia: Saunders; 2012. p. 1023–5.
6. Kilic A, Schuchert MJ, Awais O, et al. Surgical management of epiphrenic diverticula in the minimally invasive era. JSLS 2009;13:160–4.
7. Marano L, Reda G, Porfidia R, et al. Large symptomatic gastric diverticula: two case reports and a brief review of literature. World J Gastroenterol 2013;19: 6114–7.
8. Mohan P, Ananthavadivelu M, Venkataraman J. Gastric diverticulum. CMAJ 2010; 182:E226.
9. Oukachbi N, Brouzes S. Management of complicated duodenal diverticula. J Visc Surg 2013;150:173–9.
10. Martinez-Cecilia D, Arjona-Sanchez A, Gomez-Alvarez M, et al. Conservative management of perforated duodenal diverticulum: a case report and review of the literature. World J Gastroenterol 2008;14:1949–51.
11. Choi JJ, Ogunjemilusi O, Divino CM. Diagnosis and management of diverticula in the jejunum and ileum. Am Surg 2013;79(1):108–10.
12. Pepper VK, Stanfill AB, Pearl RH. Diagnosis and management of pediatric appendicitis, intussusception, and Meckel diverticulum. Surg Clin North Am 2012;92:505–26.
13. Olson DE, Kim Y, Donnelly LF. CT findings in children with Meckel diverticulum. Pediatr Radiol 2009;39:659–63.
14. Tseng Y, Yang YJ. Clinical and diagnostic relevance of Meckel's diverticulum in children. Eur J Pediatr 2009;168:1519–23.
15. Sinha CK, Pallewatte A, Easty M, et al. Meckel's scan in children: a review of 183 cases referred to two paediatric surgery specialist centres over 18 years. Pediatr Surg Int 2013;29:511–7.
16. Lin S, Suhocki PV, Ludwig KA, et al. Gastrointestinal bleeding in adult patients with Meckel's diverticulum: the role of technetium 99m pertechnetate scan. South Med J 2002;95:1338.
17. Zani A, Eaton S, Rees CM, et al. Incidentally detected Meckel diverticulum: to resect or not to resect? Ann Surg 2008;247:276–81.
18. Park JJ, Wolff BG, Tollefson MK, et al. Meckel diverticulum: the Mayo Clinic experience with 1476 patients (1950-2002). Ann Surg 2005;241:529–33.
19. Weizman AV, Nguyen GC. Diverticular disease: epidemiology and management. Can J Gastroenterol 2011;25:385–9.
20. Fry RD, Mahmoud NN, Maron DJ, et al. Colon and rectum. In: Townsend CM Jr, Beauchamp D, editors. Townsend: Sabiston textbook of surgery. 19th edition. Philadelphia: Saunders; 2012. p. 1309–14.
21. Peer AF, Sandler RS, Ahnen DJ, et al. Constipation and a low-fiber diet are not associated with diverticulosis. Clin Gastroenterol Hepatol 2013;11(12):1622–7.

22. Aldoori WH, Giovannucci EL, Rimm EB, et al. A prospective study of diet and the risk of symptomatic diverticular disease in men. Am J Clin Nutr 1994;60(5):757.

23. Wong SK, Ho YH, Leong AP, et al. Clinical behavior of complicated right-sided and left-sided diverticulosis. Dis Colon Rectum 1997;40:344–8.

24. Strate LL. Lower GI bleeding: epidemiology and diagnosis. Gastroenterol Clin North Am 2005;34:643–4.

25. Morris AM, Rogenbogen SE, Hardiman KM, et al. Sigmoid diverticulitis: a systematic review. JAMA 2014;311:287–97.

26. Suzman MS, Talmor M, Jennis R, et al. Accurate localization and surgical management of active lower gastrointestinal hemorrhage with technetium-labeled erythrocyte scintigraphy. Ann Surg 1996;224(1):29–36.

27. Wilkins T, Baird C, Pearson AN. Diverticular bleeding. Am Fam Physician 2009; 80(9):977–83.

28. Shahedi K, Fuller G, Bolus R, et al. Long-term risk of acute diverticulitis among patients with incidental diverticulosis found during colonoscopy. Clin Gastroenterol Hepatol 2013;11:1609–13.

29. Laméris W, van Randen A, Bipat S, et al. Graded compression ultrasonography and computed tomography in acute colonic diverticulitis: meta-analysis of test accuracy. Eur Radiol 2008;18:2498–511.

30. Jacobs DO. Clinical practice. Diverticulitis. N Engl J Med 2007;357:2057–66.

31. Sartelli M, Catena F, Ansaloni L, et al. WSES guidelines for the management of acute left sided colonic diverticulitis in the emergency setting. World J Emerg Surg 2016;11:37, eCollection 2016.

32. Buckley O, Geoghegan T, O'Riordain DS, et al. Computed tomography in the imaging of colonic diverticulitis. Clin Radiol 2004;59(11):977–83.

33. Janes SE, Meagher A, Frizelle FA. Management of diverticulitis. BMJ 2006;332: 271–5.

Irritable Bowel Syndrome
Epidemiology, Pathophysiology, Diagnosis, and Treatment

Dean Nathanial Defrees, MD[a,1], Justin Bailey, MD[b,c,*]

KEYWORDS

- Irritable bowel syndrome • IBS • Rome IV

KEY POINTS

- Irritable bowel syndrome is the most common functional gastrointestinal disorder.
- Symptom onset is commonly seen in early adulthood and has a female predominance.
- It has been proposed that the condition is a response to alteration in the complex interaction between the gut and nervous system.
- Diagnosis is based on clinical guidelines as defined by the recently updated Rome IV criteria.
- A variety of effective treatment options exist, including dietary modification, pharmacologic, and behavioral.

INTRODUCTION

Irritable bowel syndrome (IBS) is a common medical condition characterized by chronic, recurrent, abdominal pain and discomfort, and altered bowel habits that occur in the absence of other organic gastrointestinal (GI) disease. The diagnosis is based on the recently updated Rome IV criteria. IBS is characterized as a functional GI disorder (FGD). The underlying cause is still being defined but is thought to be multifactorial. Many treatments have been proposed, depending on the manifestation of symptoms, with variable efficacy. For many patients with IBS, quality of life is impaired and utilization of health care is increased.

The authors have nothing to disclose.
[a] Family Medicine, St. Luke's Eastern Oregon Medical Associates, 3950 17th Street, Baker City, OR 97814, USA; [b] Department of Family Medicine, University of Washington School of Medicine, Seattle, WA 98125, USA; [c] Department of Family Medicine, Family Medicine Residency of Idaho, 777 North Raymond Street, Boise, ID 83702, USA
[1] Present address: 777 North Raymond Street, Boise, ID 83702.
* Corresponding author. Family Medicine Residency of Idaho, 777 North Raymond Street, Boise, ID 83702.
E-mail address: justin.bailey@fmridaho.org

CONTENT

Epidemiology

Worldwide prevalence of IBS is 10% to 15%.[1] IBS is frequently encountered in primary care and gastroenterology practices. It is the most commonly diagnosed GI disorder. It encompasses 25% to 50% of all referrals to gastroenterologists and is second only to the common cold for the number of days of work missed.[2] IBS often manifests in childhood, though peak prevalence seems to be in early adulthood. Women are affected in a 2:1 ratio to men and up to half of those afflicted seek medical care.[3,4]

Pathophysiology

FGDs are defined as common disorders characterized by persistent and recurring GI symptoms that are not caused by structural or biochemical abnormalities. Of the FGDs, IBS is most common in a group that includes dyspepsia, nausea, vomiting disorders, and proctalgia fugax.

The cause IBS is multifactorial and not completely elucidated. Several recent studies have led to new and novel hypotheses about the pathophysiology of IBS (**Box 1**). These hypotheses have led to the development of various therapeutic options. Often explained as a brain-gut disorder, it is understood that a complex interplay between the GI system and central nervous system leads to symptoms. Observation suggests that psychosocial stressors often precede the expression of symptoms and improvement is seen with therapies directed at the central nervous system.[5]

Inciting factors leading to disruption in GI motor and sensory function may include irritation from products of digestion, prior gastroenteritis, endogenous irritants, alteration in the gut microbiome, mucosal immune activation, food intolerance, and increased mucosal permeability. These underlying disruptions lead to symptoms of discomfort, altered gut motility, and change in bowel habits. Genetic factors may play a role in development of condition.[18]

Diagnosis

To standardize the diagnosis of FGDs, diagnostic criteria have been developed; the most widely used is the Rome criteria. The first iteration of the Rome criteria was proposed in the 1980s and has since been updated 3 times, most recently in 2016 with the Rome IV criteria. The Rome IV criteria updates and simplifies the widely used Rome III criteria and can be applied to a variety of patient populations. A comparison between the 2 criteria sets is explained in **Table 1**.

Diagnosing IBS with the Rome IV criteria necessitates that the patient have symptoms of recurrent abdominal pain on average at least of 1 day per week for the previous 3 months, with symptom onset at least 6 months before presentation. The criteria also necessitate that the patient have abdominal pain in association with at least 2 of the following:

1. Defecation (either improvement or worsening of pain)
2. Change in stool frequency
3. Change in stool form (appearance).[4]

Specific subtypes of IBS often drive treatment and care should be taken to classify patient symptoms into constipation predominant (IBS-C), diarrhea predominant (IBS-D), mixed (IBS-M), or unclassified (IBS-U). IBS-C is defined as having more than 25% of bowel movements classified as Bristol Stool Form Scale (BSFS) 1 or 2, with less than 25% of stools categorized as BSFS 6 or 7. IBS-D is classified as having more than 25% of stools categorized as BSFS 6 or 7, less than 25% as BSFS 1 or 2.

Box 1
Proposed pathophysiologic explanations about the cause of irritable bowel syndrome

Dysregulation of gut motility
  Subjects with IBS received a lipid perfusion (to simulate food) and air infusion into the
  duodenum at a rate of 12 mL/min. Subjects with IBS had increased gas retention in their
  intestines, complained to controls, and had increased transit times of the gas from
  duodenum to rectum (IBS subjects had 500 cc of air in intestine vs 22 cc retention in healthy
  controls; saline [nonfood control] showed 250 cc retention in IBS).[6]
  A separate study evaluated gas infusions alone and this also showed delayed transit times
  and retained gas in IBS subjects (IBS vs normal controls delayed transit time 30 vs 20 minutes,
  retrained gas IBS vs controls, 300 cc vs 50 cc).[7,8]

Visceral hypersensitivity
  Subjects had a colonic balloon inflated to 3.4 cm in their large intestines. Six percent of
  controls versus 55% of IBS subjects had pain with the procedure.[3]
  IBS subjects experienced an increased sense of bloat and distention compared with controls,
  with similar amounts of gas in gut. This may be associated with delayed small intestine
  emptying times in IBS subjects compared with controls.[7,9]

Inflammation
  IBS subjects have increased mast cells, lymphocytes, TNF alpha, IL-6, LIF, NGF, IL-1beta in gut
  mucosa compared with controls, suggestive of inflammation. Additionally, gut mucosa cells
  that have increased inflammation are more permeable, leading to fluid leakage into the
  gut.[10]

Postinfectious
  A large cohort study showed a 6-fold increase in development of IBS after infection
  (bacterial, viral, helminth or protozoan).
  Risk factors included prolonged fever, prolonged infection, anxiety, depression, and younger
  age.
  Possible causes include antibiotic usage, malabsorption (idiopathic bile acid absorption), and
  increased inflammation.[11]

Microbiomes
  Healthy controls have distinctly different flora than subjects with IBS, and manipulation of
  microbiomes with antibiotics and probiotics has been found beneficial is some studies.[12]
  Bacterial overgrowth (diagnosed with hydrogen breath tests) in some studies correlates with
  IBS symptoms. Improvements were observed after antibiotic treatment, though this was not
  demonstrated in all studies.[12]

Food sensitivity
  The FODMAP diet has shown benefit in controlling subject symptoms. Additionally, removal
  of fructose, fructans, gliadin, sorbitol, and lactose from the diet has been beneficial for some
  subjects.
  Subjects who are biopsy-negative for celiac disease but have elevated immunoglobulin (Ig)G
  antigliadin antibodies and are HLA-DQ2–positive (associated with development of celiac
  disease) showed improvement in IBS symptoms with a gluten-free diet.[13,14]

Genetics
  IBS seems to have some familial trends, though twin studies failed to show a correlation,
  suggesting more of an environmental or social-learning component.[15]

Psychosocial dysfunction
  Subjects with IBS take their children to the doctor more frequently than non-IBS
  counterparts. Subjects with increased traumatic life events (eg, relationship break-ups, job
  loss) have increased IBS symptoms; those with good social support had lower incidence of
  symptoms.
  Subjects with IBS had higher rates of mood disorders (30%), suicidal ideation (15%–30%),
  hopelessness, anxiety (30%–50%), and somatization.[16,17]

Abbreviations: IL, Interlukin; TNF, tumor necrosis factor.

Table 1
Comparison of Rome III with Rome IV criteria for irritable bowel syndrome

	Duration	Frequency	Symptoms
Rome IV	≥3 mo of persistent symptoms with symptom onset at least 6 mo before diagnosis	≥1 d per week	Recurrent abdominal pain with at least 2 of the following criteria: 1. **Related** to defecation 2. Associated with change in frequency of stool 3. Associated with change in form of stool
Rome III	≥3 mo of persistent symptoms with symptom onset at least 6 mo before diagnosis	≥3 d per month	Recurrent abdominal discomfort or pain with 2 or more of the following criteria: 1. **Improvement** with defecation 2. **Onset** associated with change in frequency of stool 3. **Onset** associated with change in form of stool

Differences are in bold.

IBS-M is defined as greater than 25% constipated and greater than 25% diarrhea stools. IBS-U is defined as meeting other criteria for IBS without having greater than 25% of abnormal stools (**Table 2**).

Disorders such as inflammatory bowel disease, microscopic colitis, infectious diarrhea, GI cancers, and celiac disease can present with symptoms similar to IBS. For this reason, care must be taken to exclude these illnesses. A review of history and laboratory findings consistent with certain diagnoses can be seen in **Table 3**.

A careful history should largely distinguish IBS from other ailments. Bloating, abdominal distention, excessive straining during defecation, mucus with bowel movements, and urgency with defecation is commonly seen with IBS, though these symptoms are not specific. It is reasonable to question patients about rectal bleeding, unintentional weight loss, and a family history of colon cancer to screen for disease that may warrant more immediate evaluation. A dietary history can be helpful, as can a psychosocial history.

Historical elements that may lead the examiner to consider GI cancer include weight loss, rectal bleeding, abdominal pain, and increased age. Inflammatory bowel disease should be suspected with rectal bleeding, significant abdominal pain with diarrhea or obstipation, and a family history of autoimmune disease. Celiac disease may present with weight loss, diarrhea, family history of autoimmune disease, abdominal discomfort, and bloating. Infectious causes may be suspected in those with risk factors for

Table 2
Irritable bowel syndrome subtype classification

IBS Subtype	Frequency of Stool Character
IBS-C	>25% constipation, <25% diarrhea
IBS-D	>25% diarrhea, <25% constipation
IBS-M	>25% constipation and >25% diarrhea
IBS-U	<25% constipation and <25% diarrhea

Table 3
Differential diagnosis of irritable bowel syndrome and expected test results

Laboratory, Testing, Features	IBS	Infectious	Celiac Disease	Microscopic Colitis	GI Cancer	IBS
Anemia	+/−	+/−	+/−	−	+/−	−
Stool guaiac	+	+/−	−	−	+	−
Elevated white blood count	+/−	+	+/−	−	−	−
Fecal calprotectin	+	+/−	+/−	−	+/−	−
Fecal leukocytes	+	+	+/−	−	+/−	−
Elevated C-reactive protein	+	+	+			
Erythrocyte sedimentation rate						
Tissue transglutaminase immunoglobulin (Ig) A	−	−	+			
Endoscopic abnormality	+	+	+	−	+	−
Abdominal imaging	+/−	+/−	+/−	−	+/−	−
Abnormal biopsy	+	+	+	+	+	−
Historic identifiers	Age of onset 15–40 y, blood in stool, abdominal discomfort	Risk factors for infection	Chronic diarrhea, weight loss	More common in elderly, intermittent diarrhea	Older age, family history, bloody stool	—

Indicators: +/−, may be present; −, seldom present; + often present.

Clostridium difficile, giardia, or with fever and severe or bloody diarrhea. Microscopic colitis may cause chronic or intermittent diarrhea but generally does not cause significant abdominal discomfort or bloating.

A limited diagnostic approach should be undertaken and primarily used to rule out other disorders difficult to distinguish by patient history alone. It is reasonable to obtain a complete blood count to evaluate for anemia or leukocytosis, which suggests a different cause and warrants further testing. It is also reasonable to check a C-reactive protein or fecal calprotectin to exclude inflammatory bowel disease. In those with IBS-D symptoms who fail to respond to initial empirical treatment, serologic testing for celiac disease may be warranted. An esophagogastroduodenoscopy and small bowel biopsy should be considered if serologic testing for celiac disease is positive or if a high clinical suspicion remains despite negative serologic testing. Stool studies for infectious diarrhea can be performed if there is a high clinical suspicion. Colonoscopy should be performed for colon cancer screening in those who warrant screening or for those with rectal bleeding, a family history, or suspicious symptoms. In some instances, colonoscopy may be warranted in those with diarrhea who fail initial therapy, with random biopsies of the colon to rule out microscopic colitis. See **Fig. 1** for a suggested diagnostic approach.

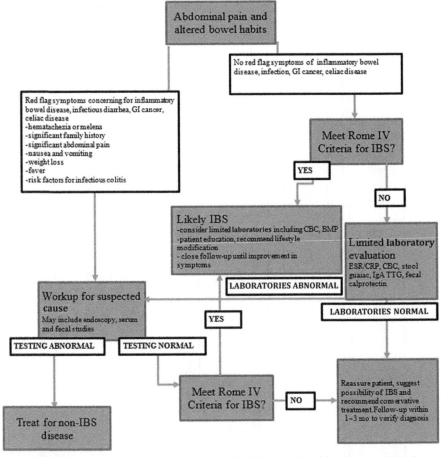

Fig. 1. Algorithm for evaluation of suspected IBS. CBC, complete blood count; CRP, C-reactive protein; ESR, erythrocyte sedimentation rate; Ig, immunoglobulin.

Table 4
Initial treatment of irritable bowel syndrome, including dietary changes

IBS Initial Treatment		
Initial therapy	Focus on removing gas-producing foods, lactose avoidance, and following a FODMAP diet. Once symptoms are under control, patients can start to add back foods (1–2 new foods a week). If symptoms recur with newly added food, long-term avoidance of that food should be implemented.[24]	
Removal of gas-producing food	Remove beans, pork, cabbage, broccoli, Brussels sprouts, wheat germ, high carbohydrate, fructose, gluten from diet. Patients who remove gas-producing foods have symptoms improvement.[25]	
Lactose avoidance	Diagnosed with lactose breath test. Individuals who are not lactose intolerant may react to other components in milk[26]	If lactose intolerant, likely benefit from restriction. If negative breath test, patient may benefit from trial of lactose reduction if other interventions fail[26]
FODMAP	FODMAP refers to foods that increase gas in the gut and which can result in discomfort. Patients following a low FODMAP diet showed improvement in scores for abdominal pain, bloating, flatulence, and dissatisfaction with stool consistency.[20,26]	
	Low FODMAP, consume	**High FODMAP, avoid**
Fruits	Bananas, berries, melons (except watermelon), cranberry, grape, citrus, rhubarb. Small quantities of dried fruit	Apple, mango, pear, dried fruits, canned fruits, watermelon, peach, plum, prunes
Vegetables	Bok choy, bean sprouts, red bell pepper, lettuce, spinach, carrots, chives, cucumber, eggplant, green beans, tomato, potatoes, water chestnuts	Artichokes, asparagus, sugar snap peas, cabbage, onions, shallots, leek, garlic, cauliflower, mushrooms, pumpkin, green pepper
Milk products	Milk: almond, coconut, hazelnut, hemp, rice. Lactose-free milk, kefir, ice-cream. Butter, half and half, cream cheese. Hard cheese (eg, cheddar, Swiss, brie, bleu)	Milk: cow, sheep, goat, soy, evaporated, sweet and condensed. Yogurt. Cottage cheese, ricotta, mascarpone cheese. Ice cream, frozen yogurt, sherbet
Grain	Brown rice, oats & oat bran, quinoa, corn, gluten free bread, cereals, pastas and flours	Wheat, rye, barley, spelt
Legumes	Tofu, peanuts	Chicken peas, hummus, kidney beans, baked beans, edamame, soy milk, lentils
Nuts & seeds	1–2 tablespoons almonds, macadamia, pecans, pinenuts, walnuts, pumpkin seeds, sesame seeds, sunflower seeds	Pistachios
Sweeteners	Sugar, glucose, pure maple syrup, aspartame	Honey, agave, high-fructose corn syrup, sorbitol, mannitol, xylitol, maltitol, Splenda
Protein	Fish, chicken, turkey, eggs, meat	
Oils	Olive and canola oil, olives, small amount avocado	

Table 5
Symptomatic treatment of constipation predominant irritable bowel syndrome

IBD-C Constipation Variant Specific Treatment	Dose	Mechanism of Action	Benefit, Harm, Cost per Month
Goal: regular bowel movements	Goal: 1 easy to pass bowel movement a day		
Nonsoluble fiber	25–30 g a day	Stool softening	May be beneficial in IBD-C only, in reducing constipation. Not beneficial in IBS compared with placebo for abdominal pain or bloating and generalized IBS symptoms[22] $5–10
Soluble fiber			No benefit
PEG 3350	17 g qd–qid (titrate to goal)	Increases stool water retention	Improves symptomatic constipation but not, abdominal bloating or pain[21] $12
Lubiprostone	8 mcg po bid	Activates chloride channels, increasing fluid secretion and gut mobility	Subjects had increased satisfaction with stooling (18% vs 10% placebo of patients who reported satisfied or very satisfied with stopping pattern) Number need to treat (NNT) = 12.5[27] $300
Linaclotide	290 mcg po qd	Activates guanylate cyclase-C, stimulating cGMP production to increase fluid secretion and mobility	Improved abdominal pain, increased bowel movements (34% vs 21% placebo)[28] NNT = 7.7 $350
Water	8 glasses a day	Maintain hydration	Most investigators agree a good idea, but minimal data to suggest benefit unless significant dehydration is present. There are no documented harms[29]

Cost estimates taken from goodRx.com.
Abbreviation: cGMP, cyclic guanine monophosphate.

Treatment

Initiation of treatment of IBS starts with identifying the severity and predominant symptoms of the disorder. If symptoms do not significantly affect quality of life, management with lifestyle modification and education is a reasonable choice. Patients should be reassured about the benign course of IBS and counseled on treatment options. Limited studies suggest that exercise can be beneficial in improving symptoms.[19] Dietary changes are a cornerstone of lifestyle modification and focus on decreasing fermentable foods. The diet low in fermentable oligosaccharides, disaccharides, monosaccharides, and polyols (FODMAP) has been shown to reduce symptoms in patients with IBS.[20,21] Decreasing fermentable foods likely reduces gaseous distension, thus altering the pain response. Though supplemental fiber has long been recommended as therapy for IBS, it may worsen pain in some individuals with IBS-C disease and may be of marginal benefit in others (**Table 4**).[22,23]

Patients with IBS-C may benefit from specific treatment of constipation. Polyethylene glycol (PEG) is a safe initial treatment of constipation but may not alter the pain response.[27] If constipation symptoms persist or if the patient is unable to tolerate PEG, the addition of lubiprostone or linaclotide is reasonable (**Table 5**).

IBS-D disease is often treated with preprandial loperamide, which has been shown to the decrease number of loose bowel movements but may not alter abdominal discomfort.[30] Patients who fail loperamide alone may additionally benefit from bile acid sequestrants such as cholestyramine.[31] Bile acid sequestration impairment is a likely mechanism for symptomatology in some patients. Female patients who fail other therapy for severe IBS-D symptoms may benefit from treatment with 5-hydroxytryptamine (5-HT) type 3 antagonists such as alosetron, or ondansetron[3,32] (**Table 6**).

Symptomatic treatment of abdominal pain in IBS, regardless of subtype may be accomplished with several classes of medication. Antispasmodics, including dicyclomine and hyoscyamine, can be dosed on an as-needed basis and have been shown to be beneficial in short-term symptom relief. Peppermint oil, which has antispasmodic activity, has been shown to provide significant symptom relief but may exacerbate heartburn (**Table 7**).[22]

Tricyclic antidepressants are the best studied antidepressant to improve IBS symptoms, including pain, and may improve slow colonic transit times and diarrheal symptoms. Selective serotonin reuptake inhibitors have also been shown to improve symptoms over placebo, while serotonin and norepinephrine reuptake inhibitors have little evidence to support their use.[22] Of complementary therapies, cognitive behavioral therapy and exercise are the most likely to be of benefit and help patients reduce and manage pain symptoms[38–43] (**Table 8**).

Treatment of bloating and discomfort may be accomplished through alteration of disrupted bowel flora. To this end, probiotics may be beneficial in reducing symptoms though it is unclear which products or strains of bacteria are best recommended. In patients who have failed other therapy, and especially those with diarrhea, the antibiotic rifaximin is approved for IBS and may offer benefit.[44–47] (**Table 9**).

SUMMARY

IBS is the most common FGD. Symptom onset is commonly seen in early adulthood and has a female predominance. It has been proposed that the condition is a response to alteration in the complex interaction between the gut and nervous system. Genetic and psychosocial factors likely predispose certain populations to IBS. Diagnosis is based on clinical guidelines as defined by the recently updated Rome IV criteria. It is important to distinguish between IBS-D, IBS-C, or IBS-U diseases to guide

Table 6
Symptomatic treatment of diarrhea predominant irritable bowel syndrome

IBD-D	Treatment or Pharmacology	Dose	Benefit or Cost
Goal: decrease excessive bowel movements	1–2 bowel moments a day		
Loperamide	Binds gut wall opioid receptor Increases sphincter tone	4 mg po × 1, then 2 mg with each additional loose stool Maximum 16 mg/d	Decreased stool frequency but no change in bloating, abdominal discomfort, or global IBS symptoms $240/mo[33]
Phenobarbital (P) Hyoscyamine (H) Atropine (A) Scopolamine (S)	A + H + S antagonizes acetylcholine at muscarinic receptor, relaxes GI smooth muscle, decreases GI motility, decreases GI secretion, P sedates	16.2 mg/0.1037 mg/0.0194 mg/ 0.0065 mg 1–2 tabs po q 6–8 h	Minimal available data Seems to help non-GI symptoms (sleep disturbances, nervousness) better than GI symptoms (abdominal pain and bloating) $1300/mo[34]
Eluxadoline	Binds to various opioid receptors inhibiting peristalsis	100 mg po bid	NNT = 10 for improvement in diarrhea and abdominal pain NNH = 16 for constipation as a side effect $1000/mo[30] Contraindicated in patients with history of cholecystectomy

Ondansetron	5HT3 receptor antagonist	4–8 mg po q 8 h	Improves stool consistency, frequency, urgency No difference in abdominal pain $13–1000 depending on formulation[35]
Alosetron (female patients only)	5HT$_3$ receptor antagonist	0.5 mg–1 mg po bid	Global improvement in IBS symptoms Was withdrawn from US market due to side-effects, then reinstated with restricted access NNT = 7 $700–1000/mo[36]
Tegaserod	5HT$_4$ agonist		Withdrawn from US market due to cardiovascular side effects[37]
Bile resin binders Cholestyramine Colestipol Colesevelam	Binds bile acids, which can cause increased stool transit times	Colesevelam 1.875 g po bid	Decreases stool transit times to the ascending colon by 50% (14.5 h in colesevelam group vs 10.7 4-h placebo) May increase bloating and constipation $50–500, depending on formulation[19]
Fiber	Bulkier stools absorb extra water	Various	Harmful, no benefit and may worsen symptoms[22]

Cost estimates taken from goodRx.com.

Table 7
Treatment of abdominal pain and spasm

IBD, Abdominal Pain or Spasm	Dose	Mechanism of Action	Benefit or Cost
Antispasmodics			
Dicyclomine Hyoscyamine	20–40 mg po qid 0.125–0.25 mg po q 4 prn	Antagonizes acetylcholine at muscarinic receptors, smooth muscle relaxer, inhibits bradykinin, reduces histamine induced spasm	Beneficial NNT = 7 improvement in abdominal pain NNT = 5 improvement in global assessment NNT = 3 for improvement in global symptom score $ 5–20[22]
SSRIs & TCAs	Citalopram, fluoxetine, paroxetine, amitriptyline, desipramine, doxepin, imipramine, trimipramine	Various	NNT = 5 abdominal pain improvement NNT = 4 global symptom score improvement[22] (Cochrane review pooled all TCAs and SSRIs in review)
Peppermint oil capsule	0.2–0.4 mL tid	Smooth muscle relaxer; reduce gastric motility by acting on calcium channels (similar to dihydropyridine calcium antagonists)	Beneficial NNT = 2.5 to improve IBS symptoms. $10[22]
Exercise	3–5 times a week vigorous	Possible increased motility, increased absorption of gas from gut	NNT = 7 for >50% decrease in pain[32]

Cost estimates taken from goodRx.com.
Abbreviations: SSRIs, Seritonine specific reuptake inhibitors; TCAs, tricyclic antidepressants.

Table 8
Complementary treatment of pain in irritable bowel syndrome

IBS, Complementary Treatment	Dose	Mechanism of Action	Benefit
Cognitive behavioral therapy	Weekly–monthly	Help patients come to grips with pain	NNT = 4 to prevent persistent IBS symptoms[31]
Acupuncture	Various	Uses small needles placed in acupuncture points to promote realignment of qi (chee) and promote the body's self-healing Heat, pressure, and electricity may be used with the needles Massage, cupping, and placement of herbs on the body is considered part of acupuncture treatments	Sham vs real acupuncture resulted in similar improvements Acupuncture vs pharmacologic therapy showed acupuncture therapy superior 84% vs 63% had improvement in severity score[38] Acupuncture equal to probiotic and psychotherapy in effectiveness[38]
Hypnotherapy	Various	A state of human consciousness used to increase attention and decrease focus on peripheral stimuli Increases ability to respond to peripheral suggestion	Hypnotherapy superior to doing nothing and standard care for abdominal pain on IBS symptom score based on small low quality studies[39]
Herbal therapy	Various Several small trials of traditional Chinese herbal medicines & Iraqi traditional medication	Reduce flatulence and abdominal pain No clearly defined mechanism	Studies generally were favorable for improvement in overall symptoms score, decreased abdominal pain, and decreased flatulence (small studies with low methodologic quality)[40,41]
Homeopathic	Variable	Based on the hypothesis that substances that create harmful symptoms in healthy people will cure those same symptoms in sick patients	68% of subjects had benefit compared with 52% taking placebo on global symptom scale (3 low quality randomized controlled trials showed small benefit)[42]
Exercise (see **Table 7**)			

Table 9
Treatment of bloating in irritable bowel syndrome

IBS, Bloating	Dose	Mechanism of Action	Benefit or Cost
Probiotics	Various doses and concentrations (difficult to conduct meta-analysis due to lack of standardization)	Repopulate the gut with more efficient bacteria	B infantilis 35,624, Lactobacillus, Streptococcus in various combinations most effective in IBS NNT = 4 to prevent worsening global IBS symptoms[43,44] Most effective in reducing symptoms of bloating[45] Not effective in reducing overall IBS symptoms[45]
Prebiotics	Various	Predigested food	Not effective[45]
Rifaximin	550 mg po tid × 14 d (may repeat twice for recurrent disease)	Presumed decrease in gas-producing bacteria	NNT = 11 for improvement in IBS symptom score NNT = 9 for improvement in bloating Effective diminishes after medication is discontinued[46] $2000 Beneficial in IBD-D
Neomycin	500 mg po bid × 14 d	Presumed decrease in gas-producing bacteria	NNT = 3 for improvement in IBS composite score NNT = 7 for improvement in constipation symptoms[47] (beneficial in IBD-C)
FODMAP	See previous table	Decreases fermentable gas-producing foods	Following FODMAP diet improved overall combined symptom score by 50%, increased quality of life, and decreased frequency of pain No change in severity of pain or bloating[20]

Cost estimates taken from goodRx.com.
Data from Thabane M, Kottachchi DT, Marshall JK. Systematic review and meta-analysis: the incidence and prognosis of post-infectious irritable bowel syndrome. Aliment Pharmacol Ther 2007;26(4):535–44; and Brandt LJ, Chey WD, Foxx-Orenstein AE, et al, American College of Gastroenterology Task Force on Irritable Bowel Syndrome. An evidence-based position statement on the management of irritable bowel syndrome. Am J Gastroenterol 2009;104(Suppl 1):S1–35.

treatment. Limited diagnostic evaluation should be performed to exclude other organic disease. Treatment is based on a trial of lifestyle changes and symptom management. The low FODMAP diet and exercise should be recommended for lifestyle changes. In IBS-C disease, fiber is of limited benefit and laxatives may be helpful. In IBS-D disease, loperamide may be an appropriate therapy, followed by atrial of bile acid sequestrants and 5-HT$_3$ antagonists. Pain and bowel cramping can be treated with antispasmodics and peppermint oil, tricyclic antidepressants, counseling, probiotics, or a trial of rifaximin.

REFERENCES

1. Drossman DA, Camilleri M, Mayer EA, et al. AGA technical review on irritable bowel syndrome. Gastroenterology 2002;123(6):2108–31.
2. Everhart JE, Renault PF. Irritable bowel syndrome in office-based practice in the United States. Gastroenterology 1991;100(4):998–1005.
3. Mayer EA. Irritable Bowel Syndrome. N Engl J Med 2008;358(16):1692–9.
4. Lacy BE, Mearin F, Chang L, et al. Bowel disorders. Gastroenterology 2016; 150(6):1393–407.
5. Drossman DA. Functional gastrointestinal disorders: history, pathophysiology, clinical features, and Rome IV. Gastroenterology 2016;150(6):1262–79.e2.
6. Serra J, Salvioli B, Azpiroz F, et al. Lipid-induced intestinal gas retention in irritable bowel syndrome. Gastroenterology 2002;123(3):700–6.
7. Salvioli B, Serra J, Azpiroz F, et al. Origin of gas retention and symptoms in patients with bloating. Gastroenterology 2005;128(3):574–9.
8. Ritchie J. Pain from distension of the pelvic colon by inflating a balloon in the irritable colon syndrome. Gut 1973;14(2):125–32.
9. Leavitt MD. Volume and composition of human intestinal gas determined by means of an intestinal washout technic. N Engl J Med 1971;284(25):1394–8.
10. Vanner SJ, et al. Fundamentals of neurogastroenterology: basic science. Gastroenterology 2016;150:1280–91.
11. Thabane M, Kottachchi DT, Marshall JK. Systematic review and meta-analysis: the incidence and prognosis of post-infectious irritable bowel syndrome. Aliment Pharmacol Ther 2007;26(4):535–44.
12. Barbara G, et al. The intestinal microenvironment and functional gastrointestinal disorders. Gastroenterology 2016;150:1305–18.
13. de Roest RH, Dobbs BR, Chapman BA, et al. The low FODMAP diet improves gastrointestinal symptoms in patients with irritable bowel syndrome: a prospective study. Int J Clin Pract 2013;67(9):895–903.
14. Vazquez-Roque MI, Camilleri M, Smyrk T, et al. A controlled trial of gluten-free diet in patients with irritable bowel syndrome-diarrhea: effects on bowel frequency and intestinal function. Gastroenterology 2013;144(5):903–11.
15. Mohammed I, Cherkas LF, Riley SA, et al. Genetic influences in irritable bowel syndrome: a twin study. Am J Gastroenterol 2005;100(6):1340.
16. Van Oudenhove L, et al. Biopsychosocial aspects of functional gastrointestinal disorders: how central and environmental processes contribute to the development and expression of functional gastrointestinal disorders. Gastroenterology 2016;150:1355–67.
17. Wilkins T, Pepitone C, Alex B, et al. Treatment of irritable bowel syndrome in adults. Am Fam Physician 2012;86(5):419–26.
18. Camilleri M. Peripheral mechanisms in Irritable Bowel Syndrome. N Engl J Med 2012;367(17):1626–35.

19. Odunsi-Shiyanbade ST. Effects of chenodeoxycholate and a bile acid seques-trant, colesevelam, on intestinal transit and bowel function. Clin Gastroenterol Hepatol 2010;8(2):159–65.

20. Shepherd SJ, Lomer MC, Gibson PR. Short-chain carbohydrates and functional gastrointestinal disorders. Am J Gastroenterol 2013;108:70.

21. Chapman RW, Stanghellini V, Geraint M, et al. Randomized clinical trial: macro-gol/PEG 3350 plus electrolytes for treatment of patients with constipation associ-ated with irritable bowel syndrome. Am J Gastroenterol 2013;108(9):1508.

22. Ruepert L, Quartero AO, de Wit NJ, et al. Bulking agents, antispasmodics and antidepressants for the treatment of irritable bowel syndrome. Cochrane Data-base Syst Rev 2011;(8):CD003460.

23. Hasler WL, Owyang C. Irritable bowel syndrome. In: Yamada T, JB, editors. Text-book of gastroenterology. 4th edition. Philadelphia: JB lippincott; 2003. p. 1817.

24. Zhu Y. Bloating and distention in irritable bowel syndrome: the role of gas produc-tion and visceral sensation after lactose ingestion in a population with lactase deficiency. Am J Gastroenterol 2013;108(9):1516.

25. Yang J, Deng Y, Chu H, et al. Prevalence and presentation of lactose intolerance and effects on dairy product intake in healthy subjects and patients with irritable bowel syndrome. Clin Gastroenterol Hepatol 2013;11(3):262–8.e1.

26. McKenzie YA, Alder A, Anderson W, et al. British Dietetic Association evidence-based guidelines for the dietary management of irritable bowel syndrome in adults. J Hum Nutr Diet 2012;25(3):260–74.

27. Drossman DA, Chey WD, Johanson JF, et al. Clinical trial: lubiprostone in patients with constipation-associated irritable bowel syndrome–results of two randomized, placebo-controlled studies. Aliment Pharmacol Ther 2009;29(3):329.

28. Rao S, Lembo AJ, Shiff SJ, et al. 12-week, randomized, controlled trial with a 4-week randomized withdrawal period to evaluate the efficacy and safety of linaclo-tide in irritable bowel syndrome with constipation. Am J Gastroenterol 2012; 107(11):1714.

29. Arnaud MJ. Mild dehydration: a risk factor of constipation? Eur J Clin Nutr 2003; 57(Suppl 2):S88–95.

30. Lembo AJ, Lacy BE, Zuckerman MJ, et al. Eluxadoline for Irritable Bowel Syn-drome with Diarrhea. N Engl J Med 2016;374(3):242–53.

31. Ford AC, Talley NJ, Schoenfeld PS, et al. Efficacy of antidepressants and psycho-logical therapies in irritable bowel syndrome: systematic review and meta-anal-ysis. Gut 2009;58(3):367–78.

32. Johannesson E, Simrén M, Strid H, et al. Physical activity improves symptoms in irritable bowel syndrome: a randomized controlled trial. Am J Gastroenterol 2011; 106(5):915–22.

33. Lesbros-Pantoflickova D, Michetti P, Fried M, et al. Meta-analysis: the treatment of irritable bowel syndrome. Aliment Pharmacol Ther 2004;20(11–12):1253–69.

34. Rhodes JB, Abrams JH, Manning RT. Controlled clinical trial of sedative-anticholinergic drugs in patients with the irritable bowel syndrome. J Clin Pharma-col 1978;18(7):340–5.

35. Garsed K. A randomised trial of ondansetron for the treatment of irritable bowel syndrome with diarrhoea. Gut 2014;63(10):1617–25.

36. Ford AC, Brandt LJ, Young C, et al. Efficacy of 5-HT3 antagonists and 5-HT4 ag-onists in irritable bowel syndrome: systematic review and meta-analysis. Am J Gastroenterol 2009;104(7):1831–43.

37. Scott LJ, Perry CM. Tegaserod. Drugs 1999;58(3):491.

38. Manhiemer E, Cheng K, Wieland LS, et al. Acupuncture for treatment of irritable bowel syndrome. Cochrane Database Syst Rev 2012;(5):CD005111.
39. Webb AN, Kukuruzovic RH, Catto-Smith AG, et al. Hypnotherapy for treatment of irritable bowel syndrome. Cochrane Database Syst Rev 2007;(4):CD005110.
40. Ko SJ, Han G, Kim SK, et al. Effect of Korean Herbal Medicine combined with a probiotic mixture on Diarrhea-Dominant Irritable Bowel Syndrome: a double-blind, randomized, placebo-controlled trial. Evid Based Complement Alternat Med 2013;2013:10.
41. Sahib AS. Treatment of irritable bowel syndrome using a selected herbal combination of Iraqi folk medicines. J Ethnopharmacol 2013;148(3):1008–12.
42. Peckham EJ, Nelson EA, Greenhalgh J, et al. Homeopath for treatment of irritable bowel syndrome. Cochrane Database Syst Rev 2013;(11):CD009710.
43. Kim HJ, Camilleri M, McKinzie S, et al. A randomized controlled trial of a probiotic, VSL#3, on gut transit and symptoms in diarrhoea-predominant irritable bowel syndrome. Aliment Pharmacol Ther 2003;17(7):895–904.
44. Brenner DM, Moeller MJ, Chey WD, et al. The utility of probiotics in the treatment of irritable bowel syndrome: a systematic review. Am J Gastroenterol 2009; 104(4):1033.
45. Guandalini S. Are probiotics or prebiotics useful in pediatric Irritable Bowel Syndrome or Inflammatory Bowel Disease? Front Med (Lausanne) 2014;1:23.
46. Pimentel M, Lembo A, Chey WD, et al, TARGET Study Group. Rifaximin therapy for patients with irritable bowel syndrome without constipation. N Engl J Med 2011;364(1):22–32.
47. Pimentel M, Chatterjee S, Chow EJ, et al. Neomycin improves constipation-predominant irritable bowel syndrome in a fashion that is dependent on the presence of methane gas: subanalysis of a double-blind randomized controlled study. Dig Dis Sci 2006;51(8):1297–301.

An Update on Inflammatory Bowel Disease

Tomoko Sairenji, MD, MS[a],*, Kimberly L. Collins, MD[b],
David V. Evans, MD[a]

KEYWORDS

- Inflammatory bowel disease • Ulcerative colitis • Crohn disease • Diagnosis
- Treatment • Special populations • Pediatric patients • Elderly patients

KEY POINTS

- Incidence and prevalence of inflammatory bowel disease (IBD) is increasing worldwide, and is often diagnosed during the most productive years of adulthood, greatly impacting all aspects of life.
- Diagnosis of IBD relies on a combination of history, physical examination, laboratory testing, and endoscopy with biopsy (the gold standard for diagnosis and differentiation of IBD).
- Treatment goals for IBD are to minimize symptoms, improve quality of life, and minimize progression and complications of disease.
- Ideally women with IBD will achieve remission before conception to avoid infertility and pregnancy complications of active disease. Many treatments for IBD are safe during pregnancy and lactation.
- Treatment of children and the elderly are similar to adults; however, in children, delays in growth and development may occur, and IBD can affect bone health, and psychosocial functioning. In elderly patients, there can be more complex medication interactions and side effects.

INTRODUCTION

Inflammatory bowel disease (IBD) refers to ulcerative colitis (UC) and Crohn disease (CD); 2 chronic idiopathic inflammatory diseases. Clinical, endoscopic, histologic, and radiologic features are used to diagnose one from another. Approximately 7%

Disclosure Statement: The authors have nothing to disclose.
[a] Department of Family Medicine, University of Washington, 1959 Northeast Pacific Street E-304, Seattle, WA 98195-6390, USA; [b] Department of Family Medicine, University of Washington, 331 NE Thornton Place, Seattle, WA 98125, USA
* Corresponding author.
E-mail address: sairenji@uw.edu

Prim Care Clin Office Pract 44 (2017) 673–692
http://dx.doi.org/10.1016/j.pop.2017.07.010
0095-4543/17/© 2017 Elsevier Inc. All rights reserved.

to 10% of IBD falls into the ill-defined category of indeterminate colitis.[1,2] This term was initially used by pathologists for severe colitis that had features of both diseases, making it difficult to definitively distinguish Crohn colitis from UC, but now is increasingly a clinicopathologic definition.[3] Both diseases can impact all areas of patients' lives: school, work, social, and family life, as disease occurs during the most productive time of life and recurs with chronic relapsing patterns. A patient-centered approach with strong multidisciplinary care can result in a improved quality of life for patients of all ages.

EPIDEMIOLOGY

Both UC and CD have similar ages of onset with peak incidence in the second to fourth decade and no significant gender prevalence.[4] The incidence and prevalence of IBD is increasing worldwide but is highest in westernized areas.[4] Data surrounding race and ethnicity are sparse, showing the highest incidence in white and Jewish people, but a more recent increase in Asian and Hispanic populations.[5] A recent systematic review reported the highest annual incidence of UC in North America as 19.2 per 100,000 person-years, and prevalence as 505 per 100,000 persons. The highest reported incidence for CD was 20.2 per 100,000 person-years in North America, and prevalence was 322 per 100,000 persons.[4]

UC and CD are polygenic disorders in which family history is a risk factor, slightly more so in CD than in UC. The relative risk of first-degree relatives developing IBD is fivefold or greater.[6] Some genes may be common to both diseases, as cases of CD and UC can occur within the same family.[7] Earlier disease onset in children of parents (genetic anticipation) occurs in both diseases but the tendency is stronger in UC.[8,9] Environmental priming with triggering events are involved in manifestation of both diseases.[6,10] Dietary changes and use of antibiotics causing transformation of intestinal flora are thought to be some inciting factors.[11]

PATHOGENESIS

Although the pathogenesis of both UC and CD is still unclear, the resulting bowel inflammation seems to be due to dysregulation of the immune system in response to changes in commensal (nonpathogenic) gut flora.[12] Genetic studies have shown that host-microbe interactions serve a prominent role in the pathogenesis of both UC and CD and involve genomic regions that regulate microbial defense and intestinal inflammation.[13]

CLINICAL COURSE AND PROGNOSIS

In both UC and CD, the typical course is recurrent flares and remissions, but stable patients more often remain stable (a patient with clinically inactive disease has an 80%–90% probability to remain so in the following year), and those with flares more frequently relapse (a patient with clinically active disease has a 70%–80% possibility of relapse the following year).

Most patients with UC have mild to moderate symptoms at the time of diagnosis.[14] Having an interval of less than 2 years from diagnosis to first flare, and the presence of fever or weight loss at the time of diagnosis are factors that may increase risk of subsequent relapse.[15] The extent of the mucosal inflammation correlates with the severity of the course of the disease; those with pancolitis overall have more severe disease. Although most UC treatment is medical, approximately 20% to 30% of patients eventually require surgery.[16] Long-term survival rates have improved since the introduction of treatment with corticosteroids and is now comparable to the general population.[17]

Despite remission therapy, CD is often progressive and requires nonmedical therapy. A 2010 meta-analysis including 25,870 patients showed half of patients required surgery within 10 years after diagnosis.[18] Another meta-analysis from 2011 showed need for surgery ranged from 18% to 33% within 5 years after diagnosis.[19] Patients with CD have an increased mortality rate that is approximately 1.3 to 1.5 times higher than the general population. This is independent of whether there is small or large intestinal involvement, or both. It is more related to complications of CD, such as colorectal cancer, hypovolemia, protein-calorie malnutrition, and anemia.

EXTRAINTESTINAL MANIFESTATIONS

Both UC and CD cause extraintestinal manifestations, seen in 25% to 40% of patients with IBD patients (**Table 1**).[20] Almost every organ system can be affected, but

Table 1
Comparison of diagnosis for ulcerative colitis and Crohn disease

Characteristic	Crohn Disease	Ulcerative Colitis
History		
Onset	More abrupt (d/wk)	More indolent (wk/mo)
Location	Anywhere in GI tract	Starts in rectum and moves proximally
Abdominal pain	Common	Uncommon
Rectal bleeding	+	++
Nongastrointestinal symptoms	Common	Uncommon
Fatigue	+++	++
Weight loss	+++	+
Physical examination		
Fever	+++	+
Abdominal tenderness	+++	+
Perianal disease	+++	+
Eye, joint, or skin changes	++	−
Laboratory		
Anemia	+++	++
Elevated CRP and/or ESR	+++	+
ASCA	++	−
Perinuclear antineutrophilic cytoplasmic antibody	+	+++
Endoscopy findings		
Rectal involvement	+/−	+++
Continuous mucosal involvement	+	+++
Transmural change on biopsy	+++	−
Granulomas	+++	+

Abbreviations: ASCA, anti-*Saccaromyces cerevisiae*, CRP, c-reactive protein; ESR, erythrocyte sedimentation rate; GI, gastrointestinal; +, degree of prevalence; −, not prevalent.

symptoms involving the eyes, skin, liver, and joints are considered primary manifestations. Having one extraintestinal manifestation increases the risk of developing another.[21] Symptoms often parallel disease activity and many of them, such as peripheral arthritis, erythema nodosum, and episcleritis, respond to the treatment of the underlying intestinal inflammation.[22]

IBD can be associated with specific disease. For example, primary sclerosing cholangitis (PSC) is strongly associated with IBD; 75% of patients with PSC have UC and 5% to 10% have CD. However, only 5% of patients with UC and 2% of patients with CD develop PSC, respectively.[22]

DIAGNOSIS

A 32-year-old woman presents to your office with 14 days of blood in her stools. It started with mild loose stools and has progressed over the 2 weeks to include frank blood and mucous. She describes cramps and urgency of stool. She denies abdominal pain. She describes fatigue but no fever. She does not smoke. She has no history of bowel issues and has not been recently on antibiotics.

The preceding clinical vignette highlights the difficulty in the clinical differentiation of CD, UC, and other abdominal processes. It is unusual to be able to determine if a patient has IBD based on history and physical examination, much less what form of IBD he or she might have. In fact, most primary care clinicians will consider both forms of IBD, as well as other pathologies, at the time of patient presentation.[23] Additional considerations in the differential diagnosis include celiac disease, pancreatitis, ischemic colitis, colorectal cancer, small bowel lymphoma, diverticular disease, sarcoidosis, and infection.[24] No single test will diagnosis UC or CD. Rather, a constellation of history, physical examination, laboratory testing, and endoscopy with biopsy is necessary for diagnosis.

CLINICAL PRESENTATION
History

Patients with IBD present with persistent diarrhea, usually with blood and mucous. Duration of symptoms can vary and tend to be more indolent, lasting weeks to months, for UC. History should include attention to timing of onset and severity of symptoms. To narrow the differential diagnosis, details of recent travel (parasite), antibiotic use (*Clostridium difficile*), risk factors for sexually transmitted infection (*Neisseria gonorrhoeae*, herpes simplex virus), ischemic disease (ischemic colitis), abdominal/pelvic radiation (radiation proctitis), and family history of IBD should be sought.[24–27] **Table 2** compares characteristics of UC and CD.

Physical Examination

The abdominal examination may reveal tenderness to palpation, mass, distention, or, in the case of perforation, rigidity. Rectal examination should be performed. Twenty percent to 80% of patients with CD will present with perianal skin changes, fissures, or abscesses.[28]

Laboratory

Tests can be useful in making the diagnosis, ruling out other intestinal diseases, and monitoring of ongoing therapy. Initial tests should include complete blood count (CBC), renal function tests, and liver enzymes. Stool culture and *C difficile* toxin should be considered.[25]

Table 2
Extraintestinal manifestations of inflammatory bowel disease

Musculoskeletal system	• Arthritis: ankylosing spondylitis, isolated joint involvement • Hypertrophic osteoarthropathy: clubbing, periostitis • Other: aseptic necrosis, polymyositis
Dermatologic/Oral system	• Reactive lesions: erythema nodosum, pyoderma gangrenosum, aphthous ulcers, necrotizing vasculitis • Specific lesions: fissures, fistulas, oral Crohn disease, drug rashes • Nutritional deficiencies: acrodermatitis enteropathica, purpura, glossitis, hair loss, brittle nails • Associated diseases: vitiligo, psoriasis, amyloidosis
Hepatopancreatobiliary system	• Primary sclerosing cholangitis, bile-duct carcinoma • Associated inflammation: autoimmune chronic active hepatitis, pericholangitis, portal fibrosis, cirrhosis, granulomatous disease • Metabolic manifestations: fatty liver, gallstones associated with ileal Crohn disease
Hematologic	Anemia, hyperhomocysteinemia
Ocular system	Uveitis/iritis, episcleritis, scleromalacia, corneal ulcers, retinal vascular disease
Metabolic system	Growth retardation in children and adolescents, delayed sexual maturation, osteopenia/osteoporosis
Renal system	Calcium oxalate stones

Data from Levine JS, Burakoff R. Extraintestinal manifestations of inflammatory bowel disease. Gastroenterol Hepatol (N Y) 2011;7(4):235–41; and Larsen S, Bendtzen K, Nielsen OH. Extraintestinal manifestations of inflammatory bowel disease: epidemiology, diagnosis, and management. Ann Med 2010;42(2):97–114.

Diagnostic tests may help differentiate IBD from other diseases and help determine which patients should be referred for endoscopy. Delay in endoscopic diagnostic testing with biopsy by ordering these tests should be avoided. Elevated fecal calprotectin is 89% to 98% sensitive and 81% to 91% specific for IBD.[29] Stool lactoferrin levels are 80% sensitive and 82% specific for IBD.[30,31] C reactive protein is nearly always elevated in CD but only 50% of the time in UC, and thus is a less useful diagnostic test.[32] Erythrocyte sedimentation rate is similarly nonspecific.

Serum antibody tests also may help in differentiating between CD and UC, particularly in cases with indeterminate pathology. The presence of anti-*Saccaromyces cerevisiae* (ASCA) is suggestive of CD, as it is highly specific for CD (96%–100%) but not sensitive (50%).[33] Anti-*Escherichia coli* outer membrane porin is less sensitive (24%).[34] Perinuclear antineutrophilic cytoplasmic antibody was found in 70% of patients with UC but only 18% of those with CD.[34,35] When tested as a panel, if one or more of the antibodies was positive, the sensitivity was 65% for CD and 76% for UC, with a specificity of 94%.

Endoscopy

Endoscopic examination with tissue biopsy remains the gold standard for diagnosis of and differentiation of IBD. Colonoscopy is the most common endoscopic test used for these purposes.[36]

UC is characterized by continuous and symmetric inflammation beginning in the rectum and extending proximally to varying degrees. There is often a gradation of disease that is most severe in the rectum and recedes proximally ending in a sharp demarcation between affected and normal tissue. There is no definitive macroscopic finding to diagnose UC. In cases of minimal inflammation, endoscopic findings might be limited to a loss of normal vascular pattern due to edema and loss of mucosal transparency. More advanced cases may show copious mucous, erythema, granularity, and friability. Histologic changes in UC are limited to the mucosa and submucosa only.

CD can involve all of or any portion of the gastrointestinal tract. More than two-thirds of cases involve some portion of the colon. IBD that involves noncolon areas of the gastrointestinal tract is pathognomonic for CD. CD macroscopic findings are characterized as patchy, asymmetric, focal, and discontinuous. Mild disease may present only as patchy erythema and mild friability on examination, with distortion of the usual mucosal vascular pattern. Ulcerations are frequent early endoscopic findings followed by the characteristic cobblestone appearance. The terminal ileum is often involved, so taking a biopsy of this area is important in diagnosis. The rectum is often spared, differentiating CD from UC.

CD biopsies show transmural inflammation. The distinctive microscopic feature of CD is the granuloma and is reported in 15% to 70% of cases. CD granulomas do not show central necrosis and caseation, as in tuberculosis.

For patients with extracolonic symptoms, capsule endoscopy and small bowel follow-through may be helpful. Capsule endoscopy is contraindicated in patients with possible stricture. Esophagogastroduodenoscopy should be considered in patients with upper abdominal or oral symptoms.[25,37]

TREATMENT

IBD is not curable. Treatment goals are to minimize symptoms, improve quality of life, and minimize progression and complications of disease. The potential negative consequences of toxic immunosuppressive and anti-inflammatory drugs must be considered in treatment decisions.

Although diagnosis of CD versus UC follows a similar pathway, treatment of these diseases differs significantly and is considered individually.

Treatment of Ulcerative Colitis

Treatment decisions in UC begin with determining the severity of disease (**Table 3**).[27] The degree of colonic involvement also plays a role in drug choice and method of delivery (**Table 4**).

Active disease

For mild to moderate disease, aminosalicylates are the drugs of choice.[38–40] For patients with left-sided disease, topical delivery is effective. Rectal suppositories are useful for proctitis. Enema formulations reach the splenic flexure and are effective in inducing remission in 75% of patients in 4 weeks.[41] For disease of the transverse

Table 3 Ulcerative colitis severity scoring				
Severity	Stools per Day	Blood in Stools	Elevated ESR	Systemic Involvement
Mild	<4	+/−	−	−
Moderate	4–6	+/−	+/−	−
Severe	7–10	+	+	+
Fulminant	>10	+	+	+

Abbreviations: +, degree of prevalence; −, not prevalent.
Data from Pimentel M, Chang M, Chow EJ, et al. Identification of a prodromal period in Crohn's disease but not ulcerative colitis. Am J Gastroenterol 2000;95(12):3458–62.

and ascending colon, oral formulations are needed. Topical and oral preparations can be used in combination and are more effective together than either formulation alone. Efficacy of aminosalicylates is dose dependent. Maximal doses should be reached before trying other drugs. Topical foam preparations are better tolerated than liquid preparations and may improve adherence. Topical steroids are less effective than aminosalicylates.

Treatment of severe disease should begin with high-dose oral steroids (prednisone 40–60 mg per day). Once symptoms abate, a taper may begin.

Patients with severe or fulminant UC may require hospitalization for supportive measures while treatment begins. Severe pain, abdominal distention, bleeding, and severe systemic symptoms may prompt inpatient treatment. Clinicians should be aware of toxic megacolon and avoid drugs and procedures that increase risk of this complication (opioids, anticholinergics, antidiarrheals, colonoscopy, and barium enema). Nutrition can continue enterally in most cases. Intravenous steroids are the mainstay of treatment.

Severe UC may be refractory to steroid and aminosalicylate therapy up to 16% of the time.[42] Infliximab, an anti–tumor necrosis factor (anti-TNF) drug, is effective in refractory disease.[38,43,44] Cyclosporine also may be used in the setting of refractory disease but is more difficult to use and has more side effects than infliximab. The anti-TNF drugs adalimumab and golimumab, the Janus kinase inhibitor tofacitinib, and the integrin antagonists vedolizumab and etrolizumab have all shown promise in recent studies.[45] Antibiotics should be considered in severe disease and with immunosuppressive drug use. Early surgical consultation is advised for any hospitalized patient with UC and for those who do not respond to aggressive medical treatment.

Maintenance therapy

Resolution of active disease is followed by maintenance therapy. The goal of maintenance therapy is to prevent long-term complications and maximize function of the patient. For most patients, remission can be maintained with aminosalicylates. Both oral and topical modalities can be effective depending on extent of disease and combination oral/topical may be more effective than either route alone.[46,47] Once-daily dosing is as effective as divided doses. Use of steroid bursts may be required for mild breakthrough symptoms but should not be used for long-term maintenance therapy due to ineffectiveness and serious side effects.[48] Azathioprine may be used for patients who do not stay in remission with aminosalicylates. Data for its effectiveness is sparse and it may take months to reach maximal benefit.[49,50] Infliximab is used for maintenance therapy in patients unresponsive to the previously mentioned agents.[44] There is no role for cyclosporine or methotrexate in maintenance therapy due to toxicity and ineffectiveness, respectively.

Monitoring

Patients with UC are at increased risk of colorectal cancer. Screening colonoscopy should be performed 8 to 10 years after initial diagnosis. Further surveillance should be done in 1-year to 2-year intervals.[27] Random biopsies should be done during these procedures.

Treatment of Crohn Disease

Active disease

The goals of treatment are to control symptoms, induce remission, minimize systemic effects, and ultimately modify the course of the disease to avoid future hospitalizations and surgeries. Treatment strategies are controversial and incompletely studied.[51,52]

Table 4
Drugs for ulcerative colitis and Crohn disease

Drug	Ulcerative Colitis		Crohn Disease		Adverse Effects	Specific Populations
	Active	Maintenance	Active	Maintenance		
Aminosalicylates						
Sulfasalazine (oral)	4–6 g/d 4 divided doses	2–4 g/d	3–6 g/d in 4 divided doses	—	Nausea, vomiting, headache, skin rash	Pregnancy: Supplement with folic acid.
5-aminosalicylate (oral)	2–4.8 g/d 3 divided doses	1.2–2.4 g/d	2–4.8 g/d 3 divided doses	—	Interstitial nephritis	Pregnancy: Avoid Asacol.
5-aminosalicylate (rectal suppository)	1g daily	500 mg 1–2x/d	—	—	Rectal irritation	
5-aminosalicylate (enema)	1–4 g/d	2–4 g 1–3x/wk	—	—	Rectal irritation	
Steroids						
Hydrocortisone (enema/foam)	90–100g 1–2 times daily	—	—	—	Rectal irritation	Elderly: Consider foam for ease of administration.
Prednisone (oral)	40–60 g/d	—	40–60 g/d	—	Hypertension, hyperglycemia, osteoporosis, mental status change, fluid retention	
Methylprednisolone (intravenous)	40–60 g/d	—	40–60 g/d	—	Hypertension, hyperglycemia, osteoporosis, mental status change, fluid retention	
Budesonide (oral)			9 mg/d	—	Diarrhea, gastritis, respiratory infection	

Immune modulators and biologics

Drug					Adverse effects	Special considerations
Cyclosporine (intravenous)	2–4 mg/kg/d	—	—	—	Infection, renal toxicity, seizures	—
Infliximab (intravenous)	5–10 mg/kg on wk 0, 2, 6	5–10 mg/kg every 4–8 wk	5 mg/kg at wk 0, 2, 6	5 mg/kg every 8 wk	Infection, lymphoma, infusion reaction	Elderly: Interacts with warfarin. May require renal dosing.
Azathioprine (oral)	—	1.5–2.5 mg/kg/d	50 mg/d	2–3 mg/kg/d	Nausea, vomiting, fever, lymphoma, marrow suppression	Pregnancy and lactation: Discontinue use. Elderly: May require renal dosing.
Methotrexate (subcutaneous)	—	—	25 mg weekly	15 mg weekly	Photosensitivity, rash, nausea, vomiting, diarrhea, anorexia, pneumonitis, marrow suppression, lung fibrosis, hepatic toxicity	
Thalidomide (oral)	—	—	50–200 mg nightly	—	Highly teratogenic	Pregnancy and lactation: Discontinue use. Children: Insufficient safety data to recommend use.

Data from Refs.[25,27,57,58,89,90,95,98,103]

"Top-down" therapy begins with potent medications such as immunomodulators or biologics. "Step-up" therapy begins with less potent drugs, often with fewer side effects. If ineffective, therapy is "stepped up" to more potent medications. The decision to use top-down versus step-up therapy should include consideration of patient goals, toleration of risk, side effects, cost, and patient compliance. As smoking is a predictor for disease severity and need for surgery, all patients with CD should be encouraged to quit smoking.[53–55]

Severity of disease can help guide therapy recommendations (**Table 5**). Patients with mild disease can tolerate a normal diet. Oral aminosalicylates are commonly used for mild disease but there is minimal evidence to support their use.[25,39,56] Because of the diffuse nature of CD, topical medications are less useful. Budesonide, a synthetic glucocorticoid, is recommended as first-line therapy in mild to moderate disease.[57,58] Budesonide has been shown to be more effective than aminosalicylates and as effective as prednisone, with fewer systemic side effects.[59–62]

Antibiotics are often used alone or in combination with other drugs, particularly for patients with perianal disease or suspected microabscesses. Long courses of up to 3 months are often necessary. Ciprofloxacin and metronidazole are most commonly used, as they are thought to have both antimicrobial and anti-inflammatory effects, but controlled trials have mixed results.[63–66]

Glucocorticoids are the mainstay of treatment for moderate to severe disease. They are superior to antibiotics and aminosalicylates in inducing remission when independently used, but can be used in combination.[67–69] A total of 40 to 60 mg per day of prednisone will produce symptomatic improvement in 10 to 14 days for most patients. Long-term therapy is to be avoided due to extensive steroid side effects. Budesonide is also an option for moderate to severe disease.

Although more commonly used for maintenance therapy, azathioprine and its metabolite 6-mercaptopurine can induce remission.[70,71] Liver, marrow, and gastrointestinal side effects should be monitored. Methotrexate can induce remission and minimize steroid dose levels in patients with CD.[72] Chest radiograph, CBC, and liver enzymes should be ordered before initiation of therapy, as methotrexate can cause pneumonitis, marrow suppression, and liver failure.

Biological therapy can be used for treatment of refractory moderate to severe CD or when corticosteroids are contraindicated. Infliximab is effective in 75% to 80% of patients.[73,74] Up to 50% of patients will achieve remission after a single dose, but redosing is required to maintain remission. Infliximab can be used alone or in combination with immunomodulators. One study using infliximab in combination with azathioprine showed improved efficacy compared with either drug alone.[52] Other anti-TNFs, such

Table 5 Crohn disease severity	
Severity of Disease	**Disease Characteristics**
Mild to moderate	No abdominal tenderness or obstruction, <10% weight loss, well hydrated
Moderate to severe	Failed treatment for mild disease, abdominal pain, fever, >10% weight loss, nausea, vomiting, or anemia
Severe to fulminant	Failed outpatient therapy, high fever, obstruction, peritonitis, abscess, or cachexia

Data from Lichtenstein GR, Hanauer SB, Sandborn WJ. Management of Crohn's disease in adults. Am J Gastroenterol 2009;104(2):465–83. [quiz: 464, 484].

as adalimumab and certolizumab, are efficacious in induction of remission. Thalidomide has been used in refractory cases of active CD, but due to side effects, its long-term use is limited. In all cases of immunosuppressive drug use, awareness of opportunistic infections is important.

Severe to fulminant disease requires aggressive therapy, gastroenterology consultation, and hospitalization. For patients with symptoms suggestive of obstruction, mass, or abscess, surgical consultation should be obtained. Hospital workup of patients with severe to fulminant disease should include CBC, complete metabolic panel, blood cultures, stool culture, *C difficile* toxin antigen, urinalysis, and abdominal computed tomography or MRI.

Treatment begins with intravenous steroids, bowel rest, fluid resuscitation, broad-spectrum antibiotics, and parenteral nutrition. Biologic therapy can be used in those refractory to high dose intravenous steroids.[75] Surgery is indicated for patients who fail to improve after 1 to 2 weeks of intensive medical therapy.

Maintenance therapy

Aminosalicylates and antibiotics are not effective in maintaining remission in CD.[66,76,77] Due to the high incidence of side effects, corticosteroids should be avoided as maintenance drugs. Maintenance therapy relies on azathioprine,[78] methotrexate,[79] and biologic agents. All 3 drug classes can decrease hospital admissions, promote mucosal healing, and limit need for surgery.[80–82] Top-down maintenance therapy with infliximab or azathioprine can be steroid sparing.[51]

SPECIFIC POPULATIONS
Women of Reproductive Age

Given that many women with IBD are diagnosed during their reproductive years, contraception and fertility are common concerns among this patient group. Fertility rates among women with nonsurgical IBD in remission are normal in UC and near-normal in CD.[83–85] It is not clear whether reduced fertility in those who have had surgery is a result of the surgery itself (ie, adhesions) or whether surgery is a marker of more severe disease.[83] Ideally, women will achieve remission before conceiving to avoid infertility and adverse pregnancy complications with active disease.[84]

Women with IBD have voluntary lower rates of fertility due to concerns about infertility, disease inheritance, congenital abnormalities, and disease-related sexual dysfunction.[83] Voluntary childlessness in women with IBD has been associated with increased disease burden but also with poorer disease-related pregnancy knowledge, which may mean that women with IBD are remaining childless unnecessarily.[84] Counseling by primary care providers can help change this perception. It is thought that children born to mothers with IBD do not have an increased risk of long-term pediatric morbidity.[86]

Contraception is an important consideration in women of child-bearing age with IBD, and many forms of contraception can be used without restriction, including barrier methods, intrauterine devices, and implants.[83] Special considerations are needed for use of combined oral contraceptives and depo-medroxyprogesterone. The data are conflicting but it is possible that the combined oral contraceptive (COC) pill is associated with a small increased risk in the development of IBD; however, COC is not thought to cause disease relapse.[83,87,88] There is an increased risk of venous thromboembolism with both IBD and COC, but it is not clear whether these risks are compounded.[83] Oral contraceptives may be less effective in women with severe disease or a surgical history leading to reduced intestinal absorption.[83,87] Depo-medroxyprogesterone should be avoided in women at increased risk for osteopenia.[83] Female sterilization can be performed, but surgical complication risks with lower pelvic disease must be considered.

Pregnant and Lactating Women

Pregnancy can exacerbate active disease, which is associated with an increased risk of complications, including spontaneous abortion, low birth weight, premature birth, ischemic placental disease, stillbirth, and cesarean delivery.[84,85] Two-thirds of women with IBD who conceive during remission have stable disease during pregnancy, and will have outcomes comparable with the general population.[85] For women with active disease, two-thirds will have the same severity of disease or worsening of disease during pregnancy.[89] Concern for the fetal effects of treatment occasionally leads to discontinuation of medications; however, many treatments for IBD are safe during pregnancy.[89,90]

Preconception counseling should involve an evaluation of nutritional status, use of teratogenic medications, such as methotrexate and thalidomide, and smoking status. Nutritional status should be optimized before pregnancy. Higher folic acid supplementation (2–5 mg a day) should be considered for those on a low-residue diet or on sulfasalazine. Methotrexate and thalidomide should be discontinued 3 to 6 months before conception. Smoking cessation should be encouraged, especially in women with CD, as smokers with CD have a greater risk of low birth weight and premature labor than smokers without CD.[89]

Treatment of IBD during pregnancy involves use of medications that achieve the best chance of remission and have the lowest fetal risk, which involves individual discussions about risk-benefits.[89] Providers should consider consultation with a gastroenterologist or perinatal specialist in managing pregnant women with IBD, especially those with active disease, but general knowledge about safety and classes of medications can help primary care providers guide patients.

Antibiotics and steroids are low risk during pregnancy.[90] Metronidazole and ciprofloxacin should be avoided in the first trimester, although recent data show that these antibiotics may be safer in pregnancy than previously thought.[89,90] Association between steroid use and cleft palate has not been confirmed in more recent studies; but steroid use may increase the risk of gestational diabetes and low birth weight with use during pregnancy.[90]

Aminosalicylates, with the possible exception of Asacol, are also safe during pregnancy. Asacol, due to coating with dibutyl phthalate, may confer a slightly higher risk of congenital urinary malformations in men and has shown a higher rate of external skeletal defects in mice exposed to very high doses.[90]

There is growing evidence that immunomodulators (including thiopurines) and TNF inhibitors (such as infliximab, adalimumab, and certolizumab) are safe to use in pregnancy.[89,90] Less is known about the safety of the newer anti-integrins (natalizumab and vedolizumab). Although the rates of cesarean delivery are higher, vaginal delivery should be attempted for most women with IBD. Vaginal delivery does not affect the disease course of IBD or increase risk of perianal disease. Cesarean delivery should be considered in those with active perianal disease or patients with an ileo-anal pouch or ileo-rectal anastomosis due to risk of sphincter damage.[89]

Breastfeeding is recommended for women with IBD. Although breastfeeding had been associated with flares in prior studies, this did not occur once medications were taken and patients had stable disease. Many medications used to treat IBD are safe during lactation, with the notable exceptions of methotrexate, thalidomide, and cyclosporine.[90]

When caring for offspring of women with IBD, inactivated vaccines can be given according to recommended guidelines. Live vaccines (such as rotavirus, oral polio, bacillus Calmette-Guerin) should be avoided during the first 6 months of life for children whose mothers were treated with TNF inhibitors (ie, infliximab and adalimumab), as they cross the placenta and TNF inhibitors have been detected in infants up to age 9 months. Live vaccination should also be delayed if mothers have been on thiopurines during pregnancy.[89,91] Titers can be checked at 7 months and repeat vaccination given if titers are low.[91] The TNF inhibitor certolizumab, as compared with infliximab and adalimumab, has minimal placental transfer, potentially avoiding interference with immunization in offspring.[89]

Children

Incidence of IBD is increasing in pediatric populations around the world.[92,93] Twenty-five percent of patients will be diagnosed with IBD before 18 years of age.[93,94] Although some may have overt symptoms of IBD, many children present with growth restriction, anemia, perianal disease, or other extraintestinal manifestations.[92,93] Children tend to have a more severe phenotype with rapid progression, especially children with UC.[93] Many of the treatments that are used in adults are used in children with a few exceptions, with use of both top-down and step-up strategies. In the United States, corticosteroids are the most commonly used initial therapy to induce remission in children, whereas in Europe exclusive enteral nutrition is preferred.[92,95]

Medications for maintenance therapy include aminosalicylates, immunomodulators (including the thiopurines, azathioprine or 6-mercaptopurine, and methotrexate), and biologics (anti-TNF therapies).[92,95] Surgical therapy is also an option for severe disease, and antibiotics may be beneficial for perianal fistulizing disease.[92,95] Data on the safety and efficacy of thalidomide treatment in children are still insufficient.[95] Anti-TNF therapies (such as infliximab and adalimumab) are commonly used in children and can be used for induction or maintenance of remission.[93,95] However, larger multicenter trials of these therapies in pediatric populations are needed to better understand the long-term efficacy and complications.[93]

In managing pediatric patients, special consideration must be given to delays in growth and development, bone health, and psychosocial functioning.[92] Many children with CD have growth failure at the time of diagnosis, whereas it is less common at presentation in children with UC.[94] Growth failure is multifactorial and is often related to malnutrition due to malabsorption and decreased intake, chronic inflammation, and corticosteroid use.[92,94] Children with IBD are also at increased risk for micronutrient deficiencies, including iron, folate, vitamin B12, and vitamin D.[92] In addition, because peak bone mass is achieved in adolescence, children with IBD are at increased risk of decreased bone density due to malnutrition, delayed puberty, decreased physical activity, and corticosteroid use.[92] Early, steroid-free disease remission and a multidisciplinary team that includes a dietician is important to achieve best growth potential.[94]

Children with IBD are at higher risk of depressive disorders, social problems, and school-related functioning.[96,97] Providers should assess psychosocial function, especially during active disease, and refer patients with psychosocial distress to a mental health professional.[97] In addition, children may benefit from a school plan that provides accommodations for IBD symptoms (ie, unrestricted access to the bathrooms).[92,97]

Because the risk of developing colon cancer increases with time from diagnosis, children with IBD are at highest risk for developing colon cancer over their lifetimes.

Regular surveillance with colonoscopy is recommended every 1 to 2 years, beginning 7 to 10 years after diagnosis.[92]

Elderly

Those older than 60 make up 10% to 30% of the IBD population, and one-third of all new cases. This highlights the need for primary care physicians to consider IBD on the differential and to be familiar with the management of IBD in the elderly. It is more common for a diagnosis of IBD to be delayed or misdiagnosed in the elderly, in part because of the wider differential for IBD symptoms, which includes diverticular disease, ischemic colitis, medication-associated diarrhea, microscopic colitis, radiation colitis, and infectious diarrhea.[98]

Although it has been thought that late onset of IBD is associated with a milder disease course, a significant portion of older adults present with more aggressive disease.[99] More potent agents such as immunomodulators and biologics are used less frequently in the elderly, who may be more likely to experience the infectious and malignant risks of treatment.[98,99] Unfortunately, there are few data on the use of immunomodulators and biologics in the elderly, as clinical trials often exclude older adults.[98]

Treatment modalities are similar for elderly patients as for nonelderly patients with IBD; however, polypharmacy, complex medication interactions, and side effects are important for primary care physicians to be aware. Decreased glomerular filtration rate in the elderly can affect clearance of some medications, including methotrexate and azathioprine, which may require renal dosing. Several IBD medications interact with warfarin, including 6-MP, azathioprine, and metronidazole. The elderly may be more susceptible to adverse effects of steroids, such as osteoporotic-related fractures, osteonecrosis, altered mental status, and exacerbation of diabetes and hypertension. Route of administration is important to consider, as anal sphincter dysfunction or physical limitations with administration may arise with topical treatments in the elderly, and therefore, formulations such as hydrocortisone foam rather than an enema could be considered.[98]

Elderly patients who undergo surgical management of their IBD are at higher risk than younger patients for postoperative mortality and complications, such as postoperative infection, cardiac complications, postoperative bleeding, venous thromboembolism, and neurologic complications.[100]

Surveillance for IBD-related colorectal cancer is based on the duration of colitis and is not different in the elderly. However, consideration should be taken as to whether the patient would be a candidate for colectomy and treatment if colon cancer were diagnosed and those whose life expectancy is long enough to benefit from treatment.[98]

LIVING WITH INFLAMMATORY BOWEL DISEASE

Considerations beyond pharmacologic treatment are important in remission therapy for both diseases. These include smoking cessation, vaccinations (hepatitis B, influenza, pneumococcus, varicella, human papilloma virus),[91] osteoporosis screening, psychological stress, anemia, and colon cancer surveillance for patients with extensive colon burden of disease.

UC and CD are both lifelong conditions with impacts on quality of life, which the primary care physician should assess and address in the overall care of the patient with IBD. Poorly controlled disease can have negative effects on psychosocial, social, and economic well-being.[101] The nature of IBD symptoms can make it particularly uncomfortable for patients to explain their needs or condition in public settings, and can interfere with everyday life activities.

For example, a student had to repeat a semester because he had to take an unexpected bathroom break during an examination, an adult patient had to beg to use a business class bathroom on a plane flight when there was a long line for his assigned bathroom, and a patient had to explain to airport security his need for baby cream and sanitary napkins.[101] Clinicians can support patients by providing letters explaining the specific needs for IBD patients, such as frequent bathroom access, especially for children and young adults while in school.

In addition to the everyday needs of patients with IBD, rates of anxiety and depression are higher in patients with IBD and correlates with severity of disease. Rates of anxiety and depression are modestly higher in patients with CD as compared with UC. As a result, it is recommended that patients with CD and UC be screened for mental health conditions such as depression and anxiety.[102]

COLLABORATIVE CARE

Given the complexity of care for patients with IBD and the fact that these are lifelong conditions, a multidisciplinary team of providers is important to help the primary care provider provide holistic care to patients with IBD. A primary care provider can work with a gastroenterologist who can assist with diagnosis and treatment decisions. A dietician or nutritionist may be especially important in the care of pediatric and elderly patients. Referral to a perinatal specialist can be helpful for women with IBD who are considering conception and provide support through pregnancy. Mental health professionals, including counselors, therapists, and psychiatrists may be necessary for those patients who experience depression and anxiety.

REFERENCES

1. Geboes K, Van Eyken P. Inflammatory bowel disease unclassified and indeterminate colitis: the role of the pathologist. J Clin Pathol 2009;62(3):201–5.
2. Tremaine WJ. Diagnosis and treatment of indeterminate colitis. Gastroenterol Hepatol (N Y) 2011;7(12):826–8.
3. Guindi M, Riddell RH. Indeterminate colitis. J Clin Pathol 2004;57(12):1233–44.
4. Molodecky NA, Soon IS, Rabi DM, et al. Increasing incidence and prevalence of the inflammatory bowel diseases with time, based on systematic review. Gastroenterology 2012;142(1):46–54.e42 [quiz: e30].
5. Hou JK, El-Serag H, Thirumurthi S. Distribution and manifestations of inflammatory bowel disease in Asians, Hispanics, and African Americans: a systematic review. Am J Gastroenterol 2009;104(8):2100–9.
6. Orholm M, Munkholm P, Langholz E, et al. Familial occurrence of inflammatory bowel disease. N Engl J Med 1991;324(2):84–8.
7. Cho JH, Weaver CT. The genetics of inflammatory bowel disease. Gastroenterology 2007;133(4):1327–39.
8. Bengtson MB, Solberg C, Aamodt G, et al. Clustering in time of familial IBD separates ulcerative colitis from Crohn's disease. Inflamm Bowel Dis 2009;15(12):1867–74.
9. Lee JC, Bridger S, McGregor C, et al. Why children with inflammatory bowel disease are diagnosed at a younger age than their affected parent. Gut 1999;44(6):808–11.
10. Xavier RJ, Podolsky DK. Unravelling the pathogenesis of inflammatory bowel disease. Nature 2007;448(7152):427–34.

11. Eckburg PB, Relman DA. The role of microbes in Crohn's disease. Clin Infect Dis 2007;44(2):256–62.
12. Abraham C, Cho JH. Inflammatory bowel disease. N Engl J Med 2009;361(21): 2066–78.
13. Mangan PR, Harrington LE, O'Quinn DB, et al. Transforming growth factor-beta induces development of the T(H)17 lineage. Nature 2006;441(7090):231–4.
14. Langholz E, Munkholm P, Nielsen OH, et al. Incidence and prevalence of ulcerative colitis in Copenhagen county from 1962 to 1987. Scand J Gastroenterol 1991;26(12):1247–56.
15. Langholz E, Munkholm P, Davidsen M, et al. Course of ulcerative colitis: analysis of changes in disease activity over years. Gastroenterology 1994;107(1):3–11.
16. Langholz E, Munkholm P, Davidsen M, et al. Colorectal cancer risk and mortality in patients with ulcerative colitis. Gastroenterology 1992;103(5):1444–51.
17. Jess T, Gamborg M, Munkholm P, et al. Overall and cause-specific mortality in ulcerative colitis: meta-analysis of population-based inception cohort studies. Am J Gastroenterol 2007;102(3):609–17.
18. Peyrin-Biroulet L, Loftus EV Jr, Colombel JF, et al. The natural history of adult Crohn's disease in population-based cohorts. Am J Gastroenterol 2010; 105(2):289–97.
19. Bouguen G, Peyrin-Biroulet L. Surgery for adult Crohn's disease: what is the actual risk? Gut 2011;60(9):1178–81.
20. Bernstein CN. Extraintestinal manifestations of inflammatory bowel disease. Curr Gastroenterol Rep 2001;3(6):477–83.
21. Aghazadeh R, Zali MR, Bahari A, et al. Inflammatory bowel disease in Iran: a review of 457 cases. J Gastroenterol Hepatol 2005;20(11):1691–5.
22. Levine JS, Burakoff R. Extraintestinal manifestations of inflammatory bowel disease. Gastroenterol Hepatol (N Y) 2011;7(4):235–41.
23. Pimentel M, Chang M, Chow EJ, et al. Identification of a prodromal period in Crohn's disease but not ulcerative colitis. Am J Gastroenterol 2000;95(12): 3458–62.
24. Cummings J, Keshav S, Travis SP. Medical management of Crohn's disease. BMJ 2008;336(7652):1062.
25. Travis S, Stange E, Lémann M, et al. European evidence based consensus on the diagnosis and management of Crohn's disease: current management. Gut 2006;55(suppl 1):i16–35.
26. Sawczenko A, Sandhu B. Presenting features of inflammatory bowel disease in Great Britain and Ireland. Arch Dis Child 2003;88(11):995–1000.
27. Kornbluth A, Sachar DB. Ulcerative colitis practice guidelines in adults: American College of Gastroenterology, Practice Parameters Committee. Am J Gastroenterol 2010;105(3):501–23.
28. Singh B, Jewell D, George B. Perianal Crohn's disease. Br J Surg 2004;91(7): 801–14.
29. Von Roon AC, Karamountzos L, Purkayastha S, et al. Diagnostic precision of fecal calprotectin for inflammatory bowel disease and colorectal malignancy. Am J Gastroenterol 2007;102(4):803–13.
30. Lewis JD. The utility of biomarkers in the diagnosis and therapy of inflammatory bowel disease. Gastroenterology 2011;140(6):1817–26.e2.
31. Gisbert JP, Bermejo F, Pérez-Calle JL, et al. Fecal calprotectin and lactoferrin for the prediction of inflammatory bowel disease relapse. Inflamm Bowel Dis 2009; 15(8):1190–8.

32. Lewis JD. C-reactive protein: anti-placebo or predictor of response. Gastroenterology 2005;129(3):1114–6.
33. Ruemmele FM, Targan SR, Levy G, et al. Diagnostic accuracy of serological assays in pediatric inflammatory bowel disease. Gastroenterology 1998;115(4):822–9.
34. Zholudev A, Zurakowski D, Young W, et al. Serologic testing with ANCA, ASCA, and anti-OmpC in children and young adults with Crohn's disease and ulcerative colitis: diagnostic value and correlation with disease phenotype. Am J Gastroenterol 2004;99(11):2235–41.
35. Shanahan F. Inflammatory bowel disease: immunodiagnostics, immunotherapeutics, and ecotherapeutics. Gastroenterology 2001;120(3):622–35.
36. Hommes DW, van Deventer SJ. Endoscopy in inflammatory bowel diseases. Gastroenterology 2004;126(6):1561–73.
37. Solem C, Loftus E, Fletcher J, et al. Small bowel (SB) imaging in Crohn's disease (CD): a prospective, blinded, 4-way comparison trial. Gastroenterology 2005;128(suppl 2):A74.
38. Travis SP, Stange EF, Lemann M, et al. European evidence-based consensus on the management of ulcerative colitis: current management. J Crohns Colitis 2008;2(1):24–62.
39. Ford AC, Achkar JP, Khan KJ, et al. Efficacy of 5-aminosalicylates in ulcerative colitis: systematic review and meta-analysis. Am J Gastroenterol 2011;106(4):601–16.
40. Marshall JK, Thabane M, Steinhart AH, et al. Rectal 5-aminosalicylic acid for induction of remission in ulcerative colitis. Cochrane Database Syst Rev 2010;(1):CD004115.
41. Cohen RD, Woseth DM, Thisted RA, et al. A meta-analysis and overview of the literature on treatment options for left-sided ulcerative colitis and ulcerative proctitis. Am J Gastroenterol 2000;95(5):1263–76.
42. Faubion WA Jr, Loftus EV Jr, Harmsen WS, et al. The natural history of corticosteroid therapy for inflammatory bowel disease: a population-based study. Gastroenterology 2001;121(2):255–60.
43. Clark M, Colombel JF, Feagan BC, et al. American Gastroenterological Association consensus development conference on the use of biologics in the treatment of inflammatory bowel disease, June 21-23, 2006. Gastroenterology 2007;133(1):312–39.
44. Ford AC, Sandborn WJ, Khan KJ, et al. Efficacy of biological therapies in inflammatory bowel disease: systematic review and meta-analysis. Am J Gastroenterol 2011;106(4):644–59 [quiz: 660].
45. Akiho H, Yokoyama A, Abe S, et al. Promising biological therapies for ulcerative colitis: a review of the literature. World J Gastrointest Pathophysiol 2015;6(4):219–27.
46. d'Albasio G, Pacini F, Camarri E, et al. Combined therapy with 5-aminosalicylic acid tablets and enemas for maintaining remission in ulcerative colitis: a randomized double-blind study. Am J Gastroenterol 1997;92(7):1143–7.
47. Ford AC, Khan KJ, Achkar JP, et al. Efficacy of oral vs. topical, or combined oral and topical 5-aminosalicylates, in ulcerative colitis: systematic review and meta-analysis. Am J Gastroenterol 2012;107(2):167–76 [author reply: 177].
48. Regueiro M, Loftus EV Jr, Steinhart AH, et al. Medical management of left-sided ulcerative colitis and ulcerative proctitis: critical evaluation of therapeutic trials. Inflamm Bowel Dis 2006;12(10):979–94.

49. Khan KJ, Dubinsky MC, Ford AC, et al. Efficacy of immunosuppressive therapy for inflammatory bowel disease: a systematic review and meta-analysis. Am J Gastroenterol 2011;106(4):630–42.

50. Feagan BG. Maintenance therapy for inflammatory bowel disease. Am J Gastroenterol 2003;98(12 Suppl):S6–17.

51. D'Haens G, Baert F, van Assche G, et al. Early combined immunosuppression or conventional management in patients with newly diagnosed Crohn's disease: an open randomised trial. Lancet 2008;371(9613):660–7.

52. Colombel JF, Sandborn WJ, Reinisch W, et al. Infliximab, azathioprine, or combination therapy for Crohn's disease. N Engl J Med 2010;362(15):1383–95.

53. Quezada SM, Langenberg P, Cross RK. Cigarette smoking adversely affects disease activity and disease-specific quality of life in patients with Crohn's disease at a tertiary referral center. Clin Exp Gastroenterol 2016;9:307–10.

54. Severs M, Mangen MJ, van der Valk ME, et al. Smoking is associated with higher disease-related costs and lower health-related quality of life in inflammatory bowel disease. J Crohns Colitis 2017;11(3):342–52.

55. To N, Gracie DJ, Ford AC. The importance of smoking cessation in improving disease course in Crohn's disease. Am J Gastroenterol 2016;111(8):1198.

56. Camma C, Giunta M, Rosselli M, et al. Mesalamine in the maintenance treatment of Crohn's disease: a meta-analysis adjusted for confounding variables. Gastroenterology 1997;113(5):1465–73.

57. Lichtenstein GR, Hanauer SB, Sandborn WJ. Management of Crohn's disease in adults. Am J Gastroenterol 2009;104(2):465–83 [quiz: 464, 484].

58. Mowat C, Cole A, Windsor A, et al. Guidelines for the management of inflammatory bowel disease in adults. Gut 2011;60(5):571–607.

59. Seow CH, Benchimol EI, Griffiths AM, et al. Budesonide for induction of remission in Crohn's disease. Cochrane Database Syst Rev 2008;(3):CD000296.

60. Rutgeerts P, Lofberg R, Malchow H, et al. A comparison of budesonide with prednisolone for active Crohn's disease. N Engl J Med 1994;331(13):842–5.

61. Campieri M, Ferguson A, Doe W, et al. Oral budesonide is as effective as oral prednisolone in active Crohn's disease. The Global Budesonide Study Group. Gut 1997;41(2):209–14.

62. Bar-Meir S, Chowers Y, Lavy A, et al. Budesonide versus prednisone in the treatment of active Crohn's disease. The Israeli Budesonide Study Group. Gastroenterology 1998;115(4):835–40.

63. Sartor RB. Therapeutic manipulation of the enteric microflora in inflammatory bowel diseases: antibiotics, probiotics, and prebiotics. Gastroenterology 2004;126(6):1620–33.

64. Borgaonkar MR, MacIntosh DG, Fardy JM. A meta-analysis of antimycobacterial therapy for Crohn's disease. Am J Gastroenterol 2000;95(3):725–9.

65. Colombel JF, Lemann M, Cassagnou M, et al. A controlled trial comparing ciprofloxacin with mesalazine for the treatment of active Crohn's disease. Groupe d'Etudes Therapeutiques des Affections Inflammatoires Digestives (GETAID). Am J Gastroenterol 1999;94(3):674–8.

66. Steinhart AH, Ewe K, Griffiths AM, et al. Corticosteroids for maintenance of remission in Crohn's disease. Cochrane Database Syst Rev 2003;(4):CD000301.

67. Summers RW, Switz DM, Sessions JT Jr, et al. National Cooperative Crohn's Disease Study: results of drug treatment. Gastroenterology 1979;77(4 Pt 2):847–69.

68. Malchow H, Ewe K, Brandes JW, et al. European Cooperative Crohn's Disease Study (ECCDS): results of drug treatment. Gastroenterology 1984;86(2):249–66.

69. Benchimol EI, Seow CH, Steinhart AH, et al. Traditional corticosteroids for induction of remission in Crohn's disease. Cochrane Database Syst Rev 2008;(2):CD006792.
70. Candy S, Wright J, Gerber M, et al. A controlled double blind study of azathioprine in the management of Crohn's disease. Gut 1995;37(5):674–8.
71. Sandborn W, Sutherland L, Pearson D, et al. Azathioprine or 6-mercaptopurine for inducing remission of Crohn's disease. Cochrane Database Syst Rev 2000;(2):CD000545.
72. Alfadhli AA, McDonald JW, Feagan BG. Methotrexate for induction of remission in refractory Crohn's disease. Cochrane Database Syst Rev 2005;(1):CD003459.
73. Present DH, Rutgeerts P, Targan S, et al. Infliximab for the treatment of fistulas in patients with Crohn's disease. N Engl J Med 1999;340(18):1398–405.
74. Sands BE, Anderson FH, Bernstein CN, et al. Infliximab maintenance therapy for fistulizing Crohn's disease. N Engl J Med 2004;350(9):876–85.
75. Kornbluth A, Marion JF, Salomon P, et al. How effective is current medical therapy for severe ulcerative and Crohn's colitis? An analytic review of selected trials. J Clin Gastroenterol 1995;20(4):280–4.
76. Rampton D. Are maintenance strategies underused in Crohn's disease? Dig Dis 2014;32(4):399–402.
77. Akobeng AK, Gardener E. Oral 5-aminosalicylic acid for maintenance of medically-induced remission in Crohn's disease. Cochrane Database Syst Rev 2005;(1):CD003715.
78. Pearson DC, May GR, Fick G, et al. Azathioprine for maintaining remission of Crohn's disease. Cochrane Database Syst Rev 2000;(2):CD000067.
79. Feagan BG, Fedorak RN, Irvine EJ, et al. A comparison of methotrexate with placebo for the maintenance of remission in Crohn's disease. North American Crohn's Study Group Investigators. N Engl J Med 2000;342(22):1627–32.
80. Prefontaine E, Sutherland LR, Macdonald JK, et al. Azathioprine or 6-mercaptopurine for maintenance of remission in Crohn's disease. Cochrane Database Syst Rev 2009;(1):CD000067.
81. Patel V, Macdonald JK, McDonald JW, et al. Methotrexate for maintenance of remission in Crohn's disease. Cochrane Database Syst Rev 2009;(4):CD006884.
82. Behm BW, Bickston SJ. Tumor necrosis factor-alpha antibody for maintenance of remission in Crohn's disease. Cochrane Database Syst Rev 2008;(1):CD006893.
83. Martin J, Kane SV, Feagins LA. Fertility and contraception in women with inflammatory bowel disease. Gastroenterol Hepatol (N Y) 2016;12(2):101–9.
84. Selinger CP, Ghorayeb J, Madill A. What factors might drive voluntary childlessness (VC) in women with IBD? Does IBD-specific pregnancy-related knowledge matter? J Crohns Colitis 2016;10(10):1151–8.
85. Glover LE, Fennimore B, Wingfield M. Inflammatory bowel disease: influence and implications in reproduction. Inflamm Bowel Dis 2016;22(11):2724–32.
86. Freud A, Beharier O, Walfisch A, et al. Maternal inflammatory bowel disease during pregnancy is not a risk factor for long-term morbidity of the offspring. J Crohns Colitis 2016;10(11):1267–72.
87. Zapata LB, Paulen ME, Cansino C, et al. Contraceptive use among women with inflammatory bowel disease: a systematic review. Contraception 2010;82(1):72–85.
88. Khalili H, Neovius M, Ekbom A, et al. Oral contraceptive use and risk of ulcerative colitis progression: a nationwide study. Am J Gastroenterol 2016;111(11):1614–20.

89. Bar-Gil Shitrit A, Grisaru-Granovsky S, Ben Ya'acov A, et al. Management of inflammatory bowel disease during pregnancy. Dig Dis Sci 2016;61(8):2194–204.
90. Damas OM, Deshpande AR, Avalos DJ, et al. Treating inflammatory bowel disease in pregnancy: the issues we face today. J Crohns Colitis 2015;9(10): 928–36.
91. Lodhia N. The appropriate use of vaccines in patients with inflammatory bowel disease. J Clin Gastroenterol 2014;48(5):395–401.
92. Rosen MJ, Dhawan A, Saeed SA. Inflammatory bowel disease in children and adolescents. JAMA Pediatr 2015;169(11):1053–60.
93. Corica D, Romano C. Biological therapy in pediatric inflammatory bowel disease: a systematic review. J Clin Gastroenterol 2017;51(2):100–10.
94. Heuschkel R, Salvestrini C, Beattie RM, et al. Guidelines for the management of growth failure in childhood inflammatory bowel disease. Inflamm Bowel Dis 2008;14(6):839–49.
95. Ruemmele FM, Veres G, Kolho KL, et al. Consensus guidelines of ECCO/ESPGHAN on the medical management of pediatric Crohn's disease. J Crohns Colitis 2014;8(10):1179–207.
96. Greenley RN, Hommel KA, Nebel J, et al. A meta-analytic review of the psychosocial adjustment of youth with inflammatory bowel disease. J Pediatr Psychol 2010;35(8):857–69.
97. Mackner LM, Greenley RN, Szigethy E, et al. Psychosocial issues in pediatric inflammatory bowel disease: report of the North American Society for Pediatric Gastroenterology, Hepatology, and Nutrition. J Pediatr Gastroenterol Nutr 2013; 56(4):449–58.
98. Katz S, Pardi DS. Inflammatory bowel disease of the elderly: frequently asked questions (FAQs). Am J Gastroenterol 2011;106(11):1889–97.
99. Fries W, Viola A, Manetti N, et al. Disease patterns in late-onset ulcerative colitis: results from the IG-IBD "AGED study". Dig Liver Dis 2017;49(1):17–23.
100. Bollegala N, Jackson TD, Nguyen GC. Increased postoperative mortality and complications among elderly patients with inflammatory bowel diseases: an analysis of the national surgical quality improvement program cohort. Clin Gastroenterol Hepatol 2016;14(9):1274–81.
101. Bray J, Fernandes A, Nguyen GC, et al. The challenges of living with inflammatory bowel disease: summary of a summit on patient and healthcare provider perspectives. Can J Gastroenterol Hepatol 2016;2016:9430942.
102. Mikocka-Walus A, Knowles SR, Keefer L, et al. Controversies revisited: a systematic review of the comorbidity of depression and anxiety with inflammatory bowel diseases. Inflamm Bowel Dis 2016;22(3):752–62.
103. Naganuma M, Mizuno S, Nanki K, et al. Recent trends and future directions for the medical treatment of ulcerative colitis. Clin J Gastroenterol 2016;9(6): 329–36.

Celiac Disease and Gluten Sensitivity

Katharine C. DeGeorge, MD, MS[a],*, Jeanetta W. Frye, MD[b], Kim M. Stein, MD[a], Lisa K. Rollins, PhD[a], Daniel F. McCarter, MD[a]

KEYWORDS

- Celiac disease • Gluten sensitivity • Iron deficiency • Malabsorption
- Gluten-free diet • Gluten challenge • FODMAPs • Irritable bowel syndrome

KEY POINTS

- Use anti–tissue transglutaminase IgA as the single initial diagnostic test for celiac disease in most patients.
- Upper endoscopic evaluation with histologic analysis of the small bowel is a necessary step when celiac disease is suspected, even if serologies are negative.
- Evaluation of celiac disease should be undertaken in patients on a gluten-containing diet; consider a gluten challenge for those who have already eliminated gluten.
- Treatment of celiac disease requires strict adherence to a gluten-free diet, which can eliminate symptoms and reverse histologic and serologic changes.
- For patients with gluten sensitivity and no evidence of celiac disease, consider first advising general nutritional improvements followed by gluten-free or low FODMAP diet with involvement of a trained dietitian.

CELIAC DISEASE

Definition

Celiac disease (CD) is defined as an autoimmune-mediated enteropathy triggered by dietary gluten (storage proteins of wheat, barley, and rye) in genetically predisposed individuals.[1]

Epidemiology

The prevalence of CD in Western populations is estimated at 1%,[2] with worldwide prevalence ranging from 8 to 200 per 100,000 for those with clinical disease.[3] The overall prevalence of CD is on the rise[4] and is estimated to affect more than 2 million people in the United States.[5]

Disclosure Statement: The authors have nothing to disclose.
[a] Department of Family Medicine, University of Virginia, PO Box 800729, Charlottesville, VA 22908-0543, USA; [b] Department of Internal Medicine, Division of Gastroenterology and Hepatology, University of Virginia, PO Box 800708, Charlottesville, VA 22908, USA
* Corresponding author.
E-mail address: kd6fp@virginia.edu

Risk Factors and Associated Conditions

CD is linked to HLA-DQ heterodimers DQ2 and DQ8, the presence of which confer the most important risk factor for development of CD.[1] History of CD in a first-degree relative is associated with increased risk of disease, as is history of an affected second-degree relative to a lesser extent.[6] Certain conditions have been closely associated with CD, including type 1 diabetes,[7,8] dermatitis herpetiformis,[9] Down syndrome,[10] and selective IgA deficiency.[11] Other possible associations include severe food allergies,[12] psoriasis,[13] Turner syndrome,[14] Williams syndrome,[15] Sjögren syndrome,[16] and rheumatoid arthritis.[17]

Numerous studies have attempted to identify risk factors in children, raising concerns about pediatric viral enteropathy infections and changes to the gut bacterial flora as potential exposures favoring the development of CD in children,[18] but this remains an area of further study. Gluten consumption during pregnancy, breastfeeding duration, or timing of the introduction of gluten, however, do not appear to increase risk of development of CD among offspring.[19-21]

Complications and Prognosis

CD has well-recognized nutritional complications, such as iron-deficiency anemia, various micronutrient deficiencies, and reduced bone mineral density.[1,22] Reproductive and obstetric complications are also possible with CD including infertility,[1,23] increased risk of spontaneous abortion and intrauterine growth restriction,[1,24] and increased risk of preterm- and stillbirths.[1,25] Children with CD may have developmental limitations, such as short stature or failure to thrive.[1,22]

CD carries an increased risk of all-cause mortality and risk of malignancies including small-bowel adenocarcinoma, esophageal cancer, B-cell and T-cell non-Hodgkin lymphomas, and intestinal T-cell lymphomas. Importantly, the risk of complications and mortality are reduced by adherence to a gluten-free diet.[1,22]

Pathophysiology

CD arises from immune dysregulation triggered by the gliadin component of gluten in individuals with genetic predisposition. This leads to inflammation and, over time, small intestinal villous atrophy and crypt hyperplasia in the small bowel (**Fig. 1**) followed ultimately by malabsorption.[26,27]

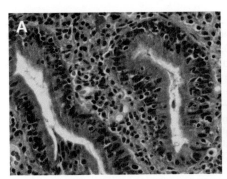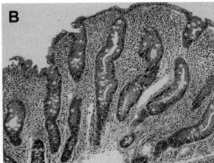

Fig. 1. Histologic changes of the small bowel associated with celiac disease. Histologic images from duodenal biopsies showing (A) intraepithelial lymphocytes and (B) villous blunting (atrophy) (original magnification × XXX) hematoxylin and eosin (H&E) stain, 400 × (A) and 100× (B).

Genetically, the HLA-DQ2 and DQ8 gene loci have been closely associated with CD; more than 95% of patients with CD possess one or both haplotypes.[28] Development of disease is thought to result from the interaction of the enzyme tissue transglutaminase (tTG), the primary identified target of antibody development in CD, and HLA receptors. This interaction causes activation of pathogenic CD4+ T cells in intestinal mucosa, which proliferate and produce proinflammatory cytokines in the lamina propria of the intestines.[29,30] The pathogenesis of CD is illustrated in **Fig. 2**.

Presentation by the HLA complex of tTG breakdown products is not sufficient for development of CD. Innate immune response may have a role in the triggering of the tTG-HLA pathway that leads to development of CD.[18,31] Importantly, most individuals with the HLA-DQ2 or HLA-DQ8 haplotypes do not develop CD. Overall penetrance is around 2% to 5% of individuals who carry these genes. This indicates that other genetic and environmental elements are necessary for the development of the disease.

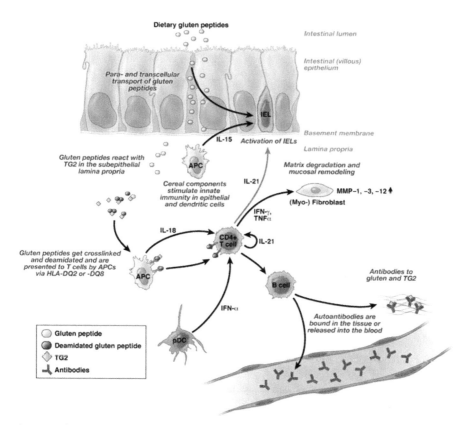

Fig. 2. Pathogenesis of celiac disease, describing the role (simplified) of the innate and adaptive immunity. APC, antigen presenting cell; IEL, intraepithelial lymphocytes; IFN, interferon; IL, interleukin; MMP, matrix metalloproteinase; pDC, plasmacytoid dendritic cell; TG2, tissue transglutaminase; TNF, tumor necrosis factor. (*From* Schuppan D, Junker Y, Barisani D. Celiac disease: from pathogenesis to novel therapies. Gastroenterology 2009;137(6):1912–33; with permission.)

Clinical Presentation

Adults

Adults may present with a classic constellation of gastrointestinal symptoms including diarrhea, abdominal pain, bloating, flatulence, nausea, vomiting, and loss of appetite. These symptoms can be accompanied by sequelae of CD-induced malabsorption, including failure to thrive, weight loss, anemia, neurologic disorders resulting from vitamin B deficiencies, and osteopenia from vitamin D and calcium deficiencies.[32] However, atypical CD is common and may manifest as iron-deficiency anemia, dental enamel defects, osteoporosis, arthritis, transaminitis, neurologic symptoms, or infertility with minimal gastrointestinal complaints. Neuropsychiatric disorders, such as headache, peripheral neuropathy, ataxia, dysthymia, anxiety, epilepsy, and depression are all associated with CD.[33] Neuropathies may present secondary to deficiencies in vitamins B_1 (thiamine), B_2 (riboflavin), B_3 (niacin), B_6 (pyridoxine), B_{12} (cobalamine), and E caused by chronic malabsorption.[33] Further complicating diagnosis is the existence of patients with asymptomatic CD in whom symptoms may be limited to signs as subtle as chronic fatigue,[34] requiring clinicians to maintain a high index of suspicion for CD.

Infants, children, and adolescents

Infants and children younger than the age of 5 most commonly present with diarrhea, failure to thrive, and abdominal distention. School-aged children (6–11 year old) more commonly describe abdominal pain in addition to diarrhea or bloating. As the age at time of diagnosis increases, symptoms often become subtler and tend to be less focused on gastrointestinal complaints. Adolescents may present with delayed puberty, short stature, neurologic symptoms, or anemia, even in the absence of abdominal complaints.[35]

Diagnosis

Definitive diagnosis of CD requires stepwise evaluation with anti–tTG-IgA and histologic analysis of the small bowel in most patients.[1]

Who should be tested for celiac disease?

Patients with clinical presentations that raise concern for CD should undergo diagnostic evaluation, especially if they have a first-degree relative with CD.[1,36,37] There is currently no role for screening for CD in the general population.[37] **Box 1** lists patients for whom testing for CD is recommended.

Initial serologic testing

The single initial test for CD should be anti-tTG-IgA for most patients older than age 2.[1,22] tTG has replaced previous tests, such as anti–gliadin antibodies, because of better clinical reliability and is recommended over endomysium antibodies because of lower cost, ease of use, and less intraobserver variability.[1,36] Higher tTG antibody titers increase the likelihood of CD but do not negate the need for intestinal biopsy to confirm diagnosis in adults.[1,38–41] Combining serologic tests for CD is not recommended.[1] Several point-of-care tests have been introduced into the market, but the limited data available suggest significantly lower sensitivity. Accordingly, caution is advised in using these tests until further data are available.[37]

Serologic testing in patients with IgA deficiency

IgA deficiency is more common than CD in the general population and can lead to false-negative tTG-IgA serologies in patients affected by both conditions. Clinicians may opt to send both tTG-IgA and total IgA from the outset, or determine total IgA

Box 1
Recommendations for diagnostic testing in celiac disease

Test patients for celiac disease if they have:

Symptoms, signs, or laboratory evidence suggestive of malabsorption, such as chronic diarrhea with weight loss; steatorrhea; postprandial abdominal pain; bloating; and/or deficiencies of fat-soluble vitamins, iron, vitamin B_{12}, and folate

Possible signs, symptoms, or laboratory evidence of celiac disease and first-degree family member with confirmed diagnosis of celiac disease

Unexplained elevated serum aminotransferase levels

Type I diabetes mellitus and any digestive symptoms, signs, or laboratory evidence suggestive of celiac disease

Consider testing asymptomatic patients for celiac disease if they have:

Symptoms, signs, or laboratory evidence for which celiac disease is a treatable cause (eg, unexplained iron-deficiency anemia or dyspepsia that is refractory or associated with alarm symptoms)

A first-degree family member who has a confirmed diagnosis of celiac disease

Type 1 diabetes mellitus (controversial)

Adapted from Rubio-Tapia A, Hill ID, Kelly P, et al, American College of Gastroenterology. ACG clinical guidelines: diagnosis and management of celiac disease. Am J Gastroenterol 2013;108(5):656–76; with permission of Macmillan Publishers Ltd: The American Journal of Gastroenterology.

---

levels in patients with negative tTG-IgA titers but in whom CD is still suspected. IgG–deamidated gliadin peptides and/or tTG-IgG are used for serologic evaluation of CD in patients with IgA deficiency.[1,37] Children age 2 or younger being tested for CD should have IgA-tTG combined with IgG– and IgA–deamidated gliadin peptides.[1]

Intestinal biopsy

Upper endoscopic evaluation and histologic analysis of biopsies taken from multiple sites in the small bowel are necessary for all patients undergoing evaluation for CD, with the exception of those for whom serologic testing is negative and clinical suspicion is otherwise low.[1,36,37] The histologic classification most widely used to describe changes associated with CD is the modified Marsh criteria (Oberhuber), described in **Table 1**.[1,36]

Some clinicians may decide to forgo endoscopy and biopsy in children with suspected CD and highly positive tTG titers.[22,40] Likewise, there is no consensus among experts about how best to proceed when adult patients refuse endoscopy and biopsy. The inclination is to perform HLA typing and if positive, proceed with a gluten-free diet for presumptive (yet not definitive) diagnosis of CD. Capsule endoscopy may be another consideration for these patients.[1]

HLA typing

Given the nearly ubiquitous presence of HLA-DQ heterodimers DQ2 and DQ8 in patients with CD, HLA typing is used to rule out CD in certain circumstances including negative serologies and equivocal histologic findings (Marsh I or II), disagreement between serologic and histologic results, patients with Down syndrome, and patients on a gluten-free diet before testing not attempting gluten challenge.[1,37] HLA typing should not be performed for routine evaluation of CD.[1]

Table 1
Summary of Marsh modified (Oberhuber) histologic classification used for diagnosis of celiac disease

Marsh Modified (Oberhuber)	Histologic Criterion		
	Increased Intraepithelial Lymphocytes[a]	Crypt Hyperplasia	Villous Atrophy
Type 0	No	No	No
Type 1	Yes	No	No
Type 2	Yes	Yes	No
Type 3a	Yes	Yes	Yes (partial)
Type 3b	Yes	Yes	Yes (subtotal)
Type 3c	Yes	Yes	Yes (total)

[a] Greater than 40 intraepithelial lymphocytes per 100 enterocytes.

Adapted from Rubio-Tapia A, Hill ID, Kelly P, et al, American College of Gastroenterology. ACG clinical guidelines: diagnosis and management of celiac disease. Am J Gastroenterol 2013;108(5):656–76; with permission of Macmillan Publishers Ltd: The American Journal of Gastroenterology.

Gluten challenge

Evaluation for CD should ideally be undertaken in patients on a gluten-containing diet because serologies and histology in patients with CD on gluten-free diets may seem normal.[1,36,37] Unless consumption of gluten results in severe symptoms, a gluten challenge of 3 to 10 g of gluten (one to two slices of whole wheat bread) daily for 2 to 8 weeks should be suggested for these patients, followed by repeat diagnostic evaluation.[1,37] HLA typing may be used to augment the diagnostic evaluation in patients on a gluten-free diet not amenable to gluten challenge.[1]

Differential Diagnosis

The signs and symptoms of CD have significant overlap with many conditions. The differential diagnosis is found in **Box 2**.

Treatment

Gluten-free diet

Lifelong adherence to a gluten-free diet is the best and essentially only treatment of CD.[1] Strict adherence to a gluten-free diet can result in elimination of symptoms reversal of serologic abnormalities and histologic changes, and significantly reduces the rate of complications and death.[1,37] Even small amounts of gluten, like that hidden in lip balm, Play-doh, and medications/supplements,[42] may lead to mucosal damage and increased complications, making complete gluten elimination critical for disease management.[36] Referral to a nutritionist with expertise in CD is highly beneficial in navigating the restrictions of a gluten-free diet and is strongly encouraged.[1] Patients with CD should use caution with consumption of oats because of cross-contact and contamination that may occur. Pure uncontaminated oats are usually tolerated by patients with CD and can actually improve the diet by offering fiber, vitamins, and minerals.[1,36]

Micronutrient supplementation

At the time of diagnosis, clinicians should consider testing for deficiencies of micronutrients including iron; folic acid; copper; zinc; carnitine; and vitamins B_{12}, B_6, and D.[1] Patients who are adherent to a gluten-free diet, however, should have recovery of small intestine absorption and should not require additional supplementation.[1,42]

Box 2
Differential diagnosis of celiac disease

Other causes of villous atrophy in duodenum[1,40]:
   Tropical sprue
   Small-bowel bacterial overgrowth
   Autoimmune enteropathy
   Hypogammaglobulinemic sprue
   Drug-associated enteropathy (eg, with olmesartan)
   Whipple disease
   Collagenous sprue
   Crohn disease
   Eosinophilic enteritis
   Intestinal lymphoma
   Intestinal tuberculosis
   Infectious enteritis (eg, giardiasis)
   Graft-versus-host disease
   Malnutrition
   AIDS enteropathy

Other nutritional deficiencies caused by[64–66]:
   Lactose intolerance
   Fructose intolerance
   Tropical sprue
   Pancreatic insufficiency
   Crohn disease
   Lower gastrointestinal bleeding
   Peptic ulcer disease
   Pernicious anemia

Irritable bowel disease[36]

Infectious gastroenteritis[1]

Microscopic colitis[1]

Lymphoma including enteropathy-associated lymphoma[1]

Allergic enterocolitis (milk protein allergy, soy allergy, rice allergy)[64]

Medications
There is no high-quality evidence in support of benefit for any medications in the treatment of CD. Corticosteroid use has been reported for refractory CD, but no trials have investigated the efficacy and safety in patients with CD.[40]

Monitoring
Patients with CD should be seen every 3 to 6 months initially and every 1 to 2 years thereafter, with particular attention paid to growth and development in children. Laboratory evaluation of serologies, complete blood count, hepatic function, iron status, vitamin B_{12}, calcium, and vitamin D levels follow a similar timeline.[36,37] Patients with residual or recurrent symptoms despite adherence to a gluten free diet should have repeat upper endoscopy and biopsy. Substantial controversy exists, however, as to whether all patients with CD should have repeat histologic evaluation. Any micronutrient deficiencies or other laboratory abnormalities present at the time of diagnosis should be monitored for return to normal as CD is treated.[1]

NONCELIAC GLUTEN SENSITIVITY
Definition

Nonceliac gluten sensitivity (NCGS) is a clinical syndrome that has been defined as the development of intestinal and/or extraintestinal symptoms related to the ingestion of gluten.[43–46] Key to the definition is the resolution of symptoms within a few hours or days after gluten withdrawal from the diet. Diagnosis also requires exclusion of both CD and wheat allergy in these patients.[43–46] Notably, there has been some controversy regarding the existence of this syndrome, because patient-reported symptoms are frequently nonspecific. There are currently no diagnostic biomarkers to define the disorder and it is not entirely clear that gluten is the primary mediator of symptoms.[45,47]

Pathophysiology

The possibility that gluten ingestion may cause gastrointestinal symptoms in patients without CD is a new area of investigation. A 2011 double-blind, randomized, placebo-controlled trial was one of the first studies to examine the role of gluten in the development of multiple symptoms in patients with suspected NCGS. This study found a significant worsening of overall symptoms, abdominal pain, and tiredness in patients exposed to a gluten-containing diet, but did not identify a clear mechanism.[48]

A 2013 study from the Mayo Clinic examined the role of gluten in patients with diarrhea-predominant irritable bowel syndrome (IBS) and found that gluten consumption resulted in increased stool frequency, with a greater effect in HLA-DQ2 or HLA-DQ8 patients.[49]

The mechanism by which gluten may cause gastrointestinal symptoms in patients with NCGS, however, is complex and differs from that of CD. In contrast to CD, studies in NCGS have shown no evidence of increased intestinal permeability or changes in adaptive immunity.[45,50] There is some evidence, however, that gluten may cause symptoms by involvement of the innate immune system with evidence of increased toll-like receptors in patients with NCGS.[45,51]

Clinical Presentation

The typical symptoms of NCGS include gastrointestinal and or extraintestinal manifestations. Gastrointestinal-specific symptoms may overlap with those of functional bowel disorders (eg, IBS) and can include abdominal discomfort, flatulence, bloating, abdominal distention, diarrhea, alternating bowel habits, nausea, and epigastric pain.[52,53] Extraintestinal symptoms include depression, fatigue, headache, rash, fibromyalgia-like symptoms, anxiety, foggy mind, and headaches.[52,53] Symptoms may develop within several hours to days after ingestion of gluten and classically resolve after removal of gluten from the diet.[53] The disorder is thought to be more common in young to middle-aged women.[45]

Is Gluten Really to Blame?

Despite the fascination with gluten, many experts have suggested the term NCGS be replaced with "nonceliac wheat sensitivity" because it is not clear that gluten is the underlying cause of symptoms.[53] Several other possible mechanisms have been proposed, including the involvement of fermentable oligosaccharides, disaccharides, and monosaccharides, and polyols (FODMAPs); amylase trypsin inhibitors; and the nocebo effect.

Fermentable oligosaccharides, disaccharides, and monosaccharides, and polyols
FODMAPs are short-chain carbohydrates that are osmotically active, are either poorly or slowly absorbed in the small intestine, readily undergo bacterial fermentation by colonic bacteria, and can cause gastrointestinal symptoms in some patients with IBS.[54–56] Because wheat contains FODMAPs (particularly fructans), there has been speculation that FODMAPs, rather than gluten, may actually cause the gastrointestinal

symptoms patients experience. This was investigated in a 2013 placebo-controlled, crossover rechallenge study of patients with NCGS and IBS. This study found that once FODMAPs were eliminated from the diet there was no effect of gluten on patient symptoms.[57] A 2015 Italian study compared symptoms in patients with IBS on low FODMAP and either gluten-free or gluten-containing diets, and found no additional benefit in patients on the low FODMAP/gluten-free diet.[56] **Table 2** describes common sources of FODMAPs and recommended replacements.

Amylase trypsin inhibitors
Amylase trypsin inhibitors are natural pesticides, or "pest-resistant molecules" found in wheat.[52,58] These proteins, although not as abundant as wheat, are prominent in commercial wheat.[45] Several murine studies have suggested that wheat amylase trypsin inhibitors activate the innate immune response; however, more studies are needed to examine these effects in humans.[45,52,58]

Nocebo effect
Gluten-free diets are common in popular culture and there is widespread concern among many patients that gluten may cause ill effects and should be avoided. The nocebo effect has been defined as "the expectation that a negative outcome may lead to worsening of a symptom."[59] Although this has not been investigated specifically in patients with NCGS, this is a possibility with this syndrome. Certainly given the popularity of the gluten-free diet, many patients with unexplained gastrointestinal

Table 2
Common sources of FODMAPS with recommended replacements

Food Type	High FODMAPs	Low FODMAP Alternatives
Fruits	Apples, apricots, blackberries, grapefruit, nectarine, peaches, pears, plums, raisins, watermelon	Bananas, blueberries, cantaloupe, cranberry, orange, pineapple, raspberry, strawberry
Vegetables	Garlic, onions, artichokes, asparagus, beans (black, kidney, lima), peas, cabbage, cauliflower, mushrooms	Broccoli, carrots, green beans, lettuce, potato, tomatoes, cucumber
Grains and cereals	Wheat, rye, barley	Quinoa, gluten-free baked goods, rice or corn flour products
Nuts	Cashews, pistachios	Almonds, peanuts, pecans, walnuts
Milk and dairy	Cow's milk, goats milk, custards, butter	Lactose-free alternatives, almond milk, coconut milk, soy milk (if made using soy protein, not entire soy beans)
Sweetners	High-fructose corn syrup, honey, berry jam, inulin, sorbitol, mannitol, xylitol	Cane sugar, maple syrup, stevia, aspartame

- Proper adherence to a low FODMAP diet ideally requires a skilled dietician
- If one is not available, online resources and mobile Apps are available
- A 2–4 wk trial will generally suffice to see if there are improvements
- Note: low FODMAP is not recommended in a generally healthy diet, it is only for diagnosing dietary causes of gastrointestinal symptoms and once this is identified, it is recommended working with a dietician to liberalize diet as much as possible

Adapted from Gibson PR, Varney J, Malakar S, et al, Food Components and IBS. Gastroenterology 2015;148:1158–74; and Chey WD. Food: the main course to wellness and illness in patients with IBS. Am J Gastroenterol 2016;111:366–71; with permission.

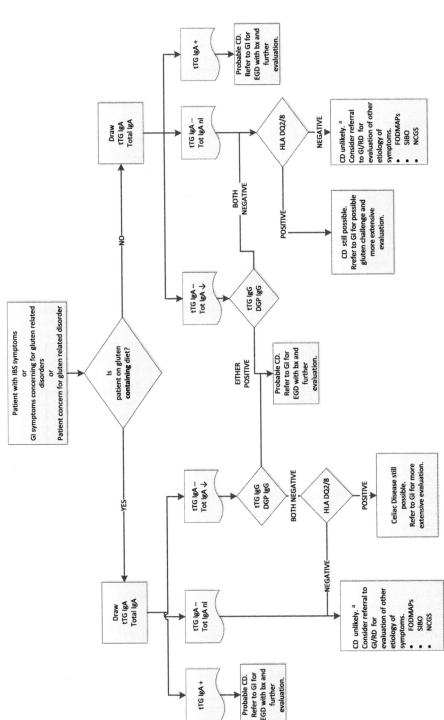

Fig. 3. Suggested approach to diagnosis and management of patients with symptoms pertaining to gluten-related disorders. [a]If it has not already been instituted, a trial of general dietary improvement may be considered before referral including more fresh fruits and vegetables, whole grains, nonfried low-fat sources of protein, and avoiding processed snack foods. DGP IgG, deamidated gliadin peptide immunoglobulin G; GI, gastroenterology specialist; RD, registered dietician; SIBO, small intestinal bacterial overgrowth.

symptoms self-restrict gluten because of the popular belief that gluten may be the underlying cause of these symptoms. Unfortunately, this can often result in significant stress, food restriction, and often confuses evaluation.

Diagnosis and Treatment

NCGS is a clinical diagnosis, because there are no specific laboratory tests or clinical biomarkers that characterize the syndrome.[60] If there is concern for this disorder (typically based on patient-reported symptoms), it is imperative to rule out CD or wheat allergy (if applicable) before evaluating for the possibility of NCGS.[46] A complex practice called a double-blind, placebo-controlled gluten challenge has typically been considered to be the best way to diagnose this syndrome. A group of experts recently published recommendations regarding a practical way to institute the double-blind, placebo-controlled gluten challenge.[46] However, the process is still complicated and cumbersome to use in general practice, and is best instituted under the guidance of a dietician and gastroenterologist.

Ultimately, it is imperative to synthesize the somewhat conflicting data on NCGS to advise patients on the best course of action to improve symptoms. If a patient is concerned that his or her gastrointestinal symptoms are related to gluten, then it is imperative to first rule out CD and/or wheat allergy. If this evaluation is negative, and if the patient has not already implemented dietary changes on their own, it is reasonable to first make general nutritional improvements: eating more fresh fruits and vegetables, whole grains, and nonfried low-fat sources of protein, while avoiding processed snack foods.[61] If there is no improvement, then there are several approaches to manage symptoms, which can include a gluten-free diet, low FODMAP diet, evaluation for small intestinal bacterial overgrowth, or other treatments for IBS. If instituting these more restrictive dietary therapies, it is key to involve the skills of a trained dietician to help patients navigate these dietary changes in a healthy and safe way to avoid overrestriction and nutritional deficiencies.

DISCUSSION

Despite the harms of delayed diagnosis including increased risk of cancer[62] and death,[63] CD is often unrecognized[3] or misdiagnosed (often as IBS).[2] CD and NCGS are related but distinct conditions that can present similarly, each with the potential to severely impact quality of life. However, the long-term consequences of CD are much more significant, making the diagnostic distinction between these two conditions crucial. Management of CD requires strict adherence to a gluten-free diet, not only for symptom control, but for reduction of the risk of complications and mortality. A gluten-free diet is, however, only one of several treatment options for patients with NCGS. **Fig. 3** provides a suggested approach to diagnosis and management of patients with symptoms pertaining to gluten-related disorders.

ACKNOWLEDGMENTS

Anne M. Mills, MD

REFERENCES

1. Rubio-Tapia A, Hill ID, Kelly P, et al, American College of Gastroenterology. ACG clinical guidelines: diagnosis and management of celiac disease. Am J Gastroenterol 2013;108(5):656–76 [quiz: 677].

2. Dubé C, Rostom A, Sy R, et al. The prevalence of celiac disease in average-risk and at-risk Western European populations: a systematic review. Gastroenterology 2005;128(4 Suppl 1):S57–67. Available at: http://www.ncbi.nlm.nih.gov/pubmed/15825128. Accessed November 18, 2016.

3. Kang JY, Kang AHY, Green A, et al. Systematic review: worldwide variation in the frequency of coeliac disease and changes over time. Aliment Pharmacol Ther 2013;38(3):226–45.

4. Riddle MS, Murray JA, Porter CK. The incidence and risk of celiac disease in a healthy US adult population. Am J Gastroenterol 2012;107(8):1248–55.

5. Population clock. Available at: https://www.census.gov/popclock/. Accessed October 18, 2016.

6. Singh P, Arora S, Lal S, et al. Risk of celiac disease in the first- and second-degree relatives of patients with celiac disease: a systematic review and meta-analysis. Am J Gastroenterol 2015;110(11):1539–48.

7. Pham-Short A, Donaghue KC, Ambler G, et al. Coeliac disease in type 1 diabetes from 1990 to 2009: higher incidence in young children after longer diabetes duration. Diabet Med 2012;29(9):e286–9.

8. Mahmud FH, Murray JA, Kudva YC, et al. Celiac disease in type 1 diabetes mellitus in a North American community: prevalence, serologic screening, and clinical features. Mayo Clin Proc 2005;80(11):1429–34.

9. Balas A, Vicario JL, Zambrano A, et al. Absolute linkage of celiac disease and dermatitis herpetiformis to HLA-DQ. Tissue Antigens 1997;50(1):52–6. Available at: http://www.ncbi.nlm.nih.gov/pubmed/9243756. Accessed December 2, 2016.

10. Mårild K, Stephansson O, Grahnquist L, et al. Down syndrome is associated with elevated risk of celiac disease: a nationwide case-control study. J Pediatr 2013;163(1):237–42.

11. Ludvigsson JF, Neovius M, Hammarström L. Association between IgA deficiency & other autoimmune conditions: a population-based matched cohort study. J Clin Immunol 2014;34(4):444–51.

12. Pillon R, Ziberna F, Badina L, et al. Prevalence of celiac disease in patients with severe food allergy. Allergy 2015;70(10):1346–9.

13. De Bastiani R, Gabrielli M, Lora L, et al. Association between coeliac disease and psoriasis: Italian primary care multicentre study. Dermatology 2015;230(2):156–60.

14. Marild K, Stordal K, Hagman A, et al. Turner syndrome and celiac disease: a case-control study. Pediatrics 2016;137(2):e20152232.

15. Giannotti A, Tiberio G, Castro M, et al. Coeliac disease in Williams syndrome. J Med Genet 2001;38(11):767–8. Available at: http://www.ncbi.nlm.nih.gov/pubmed/11694549. Accessed November 18, 2016.

16. Patinen P, Aine L, Collin P, et al. Oral findings in coeliac disease and Sjögren's syndrome. Oral Dis 2004;10(6):330–4.

17. Neuhausen SL, Steele L, Ryan S, et al. Co-occurrence of celiac disease and other autoimmune diseases in celiacs and their first-degree relatives. J Autoimmun 2008;31(2):160–5.

18. Schuppan D, Junker Y, Barisani D. Celiac disease: from pathogenesis to novel therapies. Gastroenterology 2009;137(6):1912–33.

19. Uusitalo U, Lee H-S, Aronsson CA, et al. Gluten consumption during late pregnancy and risk of celiac disease in the offspring: the TEDDY birth cohort. Am J Clin Nutr 2015;102(5):1216–21.

20. Silano M, Agostoni C, Sanz Y, et al. Infant feeding and risk of developing celiac disease: a systematic review. BMJ Open 2016;6(1). e009163.

21. Aronsson CA, Lee H-S, Liu E, et al. Age at gluten introduction and risk of celiac disease. Pediatrics 2015;135(2):239–45.
22. Husby S, Koletzko S, Korponay-Szabó IR, et al. European society for pediatric gastroenterology, hepatology, and nutrition guidelines for the diagnosis of coeliac disease. J Pediatr Gastroenterol Nutr 2012;54(1):136–60.
23. Zugna D, Richiardi L, Akre O, et al. A nationwide population-based study to determine whether coeliac disease is associated with infertility. Gut 2010; 59(11):1471–5.
24. Gasbarrini A, Torre ES, Trivellini C, et al. Recurrent spontaneous abortion and intrauterine fetal growth retardation as symptoms of coeliac disease. Lancet 2000; 356(9227):399–400.
25. Saccone G, Berghella V, Sarno L, et al. Celiac disease and obstetric complications: a systematic review and metaanalysis. Am J Obstet Gynecol 2016; 214(2):225–34.
26. Schuppan D. Current concepts of celiac disease pathogenesis. Gastroenterology 2000;119(1):234–42. Available at: http://www.ncbi.nlm.nih.gov/pubmed/ 10889174. Accessed December 2, 2016.
27. Kagnoff MF. Celiac disease. A gastrointestinal disease with environmental, genetic, and immunologic components. Gastroenterol Clin North Am 1992;21(2): 405–25. Available at: http://www.ncbi.nlm.nih.gov/pubmed/1512049. Accessed December 2, 2016.
28. Kaukinen K, Partanen J, Mäki M, et al. HLA-DQ typing in the diagnosis of celiac disease. Am J Gastroenterol 2002;97(3):695–9.
29. Hourigan CS. The molecular basis of coeliac disease. Clin Exp Med 2006;6(2): 53–9.
30. Molberg O, Mcadam SN, Körner R, et al. Tissue transglutaminase selectively modifies gliadin peptides that are recognized by gut-derived T cells in celiac disease. Nat Med 1998;4(6):713–7. Available at: http://www.ncbi.nlm.nih.gov/ pubmed/9623982. Accessed December 2, 2016.
31. Maiuri L, Ciacci C, Ricciardelli I, et al. Association between innate response to gliadin and activation of pathogenic T cells in celiac disease. Lancet 2003; 362(9377):30–7.
32. Catassi C, Kryszak D, Louis-Jacques O, et al. Detection of celiac disease in primary care: a multicenter case-finding study in North America. Am J Gastroenterol 2007;102(7):1454–60.
33. Holmes GK. Non-malignant complications of coeliac disease. Acta Paediatr Suppl 1996;412:68–75. Available at: http://www.ncbi.nlm.nih.gov/pubmed/ 8783765. Accessed December 2, 2016.
34. Rampertab SD, Pooran N, Brar P, et al. Trends in the presentation of celiac disease. Am J Med 2006;119(4):355.e9-e14.
35. Tanpowpong P, Broder-Fingert S, Katz AJ, et al. Age-related patterns in clinical presentations and gluten-related issues among children and adolescents with celiac disease. Clin Transl Gastroenterol 2012;3(2):e9.
36. JC Bai, Ciacci. World gastroenterology organisation global guidelines celiac disease WGO global guidelines celiac disease (long version) 2. J Clin Gastroenterol 2013 Feb;47(2):121–6. http://dx.doi.org/10.1097/MCG.0b013e31827a6f83. Updated July 2016.
37. Ludvigsson JF, Bai JC, Biagi F, et al. Diagnosis and management of adult coeliac disease: guidelines from the British Society of Gastroenterology. Gut 2014;63(8): 1210–28.

38. Elitsur Y, Sigman T, Watkins R, et al. Tissue transglutaminase levels are not sufficient to diagnose celiac disease in North American practices without intestinal biopsies. Dig Dis Sci 2017;62(1):175–9.
39. John M. Eisenberg Center for Clinical Decisions and Communications Science. Diagnosis of celiac disease: current state of the evidence; 2007. Available at: http://www.ncbi.nlm.nih.gov/pubmed/27583323. Accessed November 11, 2016.
40. Murray J, Scanlon SA. Update on celiac disease: etiology, differential diagnosis, drug targets, and management advances. Clin Exp Gastroenterol 2011;4: 297–311.
41. Vavricka SR, Stelzer T, Lattmann J, et al. Celiac disease is misdiagnosed based on serology only in a substantial proportion of patients. J Clin Gastroenterol 2016;1. http://dx.doi.org/10.1097/MCG.0000000000000676.
42. Sources of gluten - Celiac Disease Foundation. Available at: https://celiac.org/live-gluten-free/glutenfreediet/sources-of-gluten/. Accessed November 21, 2016.
43. Sapone A, Bai JC, Ciacci C, et al. Spectrum of gluten-related disorders: consensus on new nomenclature and classification. BMC Med 2012;10(1):13.
44. Ludvigsson JF, Leffler DA, Bai JC, et al. The Oslo definitions for coeliac disease and related terms. Gut 2013;62(1):43–52.
45. Fasano A, Sapone A, Zevallos V, et al. Nonceliac gluten sensitivity. Gastroenterology 2015;148(6):1195–204.
46. Catassi C, Elli L, Bonaz B, et al. Diagnosis of non-celiac gluten sensitivity (NCGS): the Salerno experts' criteria. Nutrients 2015;7(6):4966–77.
47. Volta U, Caio G, De Giorgio R, et al. Non-celiac gluten sensitivity: a work-in-progress entity in the spectrum of wheat-related disorders. Best Pract Res Clin Gastroenterol 2015;29(3):477–91.
48. Biesiekierski JR, Newnham ED, Irving PM, et al. Gluten causes gastrointestinal symptoms in subjects without celiac disease: a double-blind randomized placebo-controlled trial. Am J Gastroenterol 2011;106(3):508–14.
49. Vazquez–Roque MI, Camilleri M, Smyrk T, et al. A controlled trial of gluten-free diet in patients with irritable bowel syndrome-diarrhea: effects on bowel frequency and intestinal function. Gastroenterology 2013;144(5):903–11.e3.
50. Sapone A, Lammers KM, Casolaro V, et al. Divergence of gut permeability and mucosal immune gene expression in two gluten-associated conditions: celiac disease and gluten sensitivity. BMC Med 2011;9(1):23.
51. Sapone A, Lammers KM, Mazzarella G, et al. Differential mucosal IL-17 expression in two gliadin-induced disorders: gluten sensitivity and the autoimmune enteropathy celiac disease. Int Arch Allergy Immunol 2010;152(1):75–80.
52. Aziz I, Hadjivassiliou M, Sanders DS. The spectrum of noncoeliac gluten sensitivity. Nat Rev Gastroenterol Hepatol 2015;12(9):516–26.
53. Aziz I, Dwivedi K, Sanders DS. From coeliac disease to noncoeliac gluten sensitivity; should everyone be gluten free? Curr Opin Gastroenterol 2016;32(2):120–7.
54. Halmos EP, Power VA, Shepherd SJ, et al. A diet low in FODMAPs reduces symptoms of irritable bowel syndrome. Gastroenterology 2014;146(1):67–75.e5.
55. Gibson PR, Shepherd SJ. Food choice as a key management strategy for functional gastrointestinal symptoms. Am J Gastroenterol 2012;107(5):657–66.
56. Chey WD. Food: the main course to wellness and illness in patients with irritable bowel syndrome. Am J Gastroenterol 2016;111(3):366–71.
57. Biesiekierski JR, Peters SL, Newnham ED, et al. No effects of gluten in patients with self-reported non-celiac gluten sensitivity after dietary reduction of fermentable, poorly absorbed, short-chain carbohydrates. Gastroenterology 2013; 145(2):320–8.e3.

58. Junker Y, Zeissig S, Kim S-J, et al. Wheat amylase trypsin inhibitors drive intestinal inflammation via activation of toll-like receptor 4. J Exp Med 2012;209(13): 2395–408.
59. Benedetti F, Lanotte M, Lopiano L, et al. When words are painful: unraveling the mechanisms of the nocebo effect. Neuroscience 2007;147(2):260–71.
60. Volta U, Pinto-Sanchez MI, Boschetti E, et al. Dietary triggers in irritable bowel syndrome: is there a role for gluten? J Neurogastroenterol Motil 2016;22(4): 547–57.
61. McCarter DF. Non-celiac gluten sensitivity: important diagnosis or dietary fad? Am Fam Physician 2014;89(2):82–3. Available at: http://www.ncbi.nlm.nih.gov/pubmed/24444574. Accessed November 30, 2016.
62. Green PHR, Fleischauer AT, Bhagat G, et al. Risk of malignancy in patients with celiac disease. Am J Med 2003;115(3):191–5. Available at: http://www.ncbi.nlm.nih.gov/pubmed/12935825. Accessed November 17, 2016.
63. Rubio-Tapia A, Kyle RA, Kaplan EL, et al. Increased prevalence and mortality in undiagnosed celiac disease. Gastroenterology 2009;137(1):88–93.
64. DynaMed Plus. DynaMed Plus [Internet]. Ipswich (MA): EBSCO Information Services; 1995. Record No. 114570, Celiac disease; [updated 2016 Sep 14]; [about 31 screens]. Available at: http://www.dynamed.com/topics/dmp~AN~T114570/Celiac-disease. Accessed November 22, 2016.
65. Biesiekierski JR, Iven J. Non-coeliac gluten sensitivity: piecing the puzzle together. United European Gastroenterol J 2015;3(2):160–5.
66. Fasano A, Catassi C. Clinical practice. Celiac disease. N Engl J Med 2012; 367(25):2419–26.

Diagnosis and Management of Anorectal Disorders in the Primary Care Setting

Danielle Davies, MD[a,b,*], Justin Bailey, MD[b,c]

KEYWORDS

- Rectal prolapse • Hemorrhoids • Anal fissure • Proctalgia fugax • Levator ani

KEY POINTS

- Avoiding constipation through diet modification and use of over-the-counter medications can prevent many of the common anorectal disorders that present to the primary care physician.
- Rectal prolapse should be reduced when possible and can be treated conservatively in most situations, although patients with recurrence may require surgical intervention.
- Pruritus ani often has an inciting event, but treatment should focus on stopping the itch–scratch cycle that worsens the symptoms.
- Thrombosed external hemorrhoids can be excised in the office when patients present within 72 hours of onset and when they do not have improvement in symptoms.
- Internal hemorrhoids can be successfully banded in the office, although postprocedure pain is common.

INTRODUCTION

Anorectal disorders are very common among a wide population of patients. Because patients may be embarrassed about the anatomic location of their symptoms, they may present to care late in the course of their illness. Care should be taken to validate patient concerns and normalize fears. This article discusses the diagnoses and management of common anorectal disorders among patients presenting to a primary care physician.

RECTAL PROLAPSE

Rectal prolapse, also known as rectal procidentia, occurs when the rectum protrudes through the anus. This protrusion may involve just the mucosa and submucosa (partial

The authors have nothing to disclose.
[a] Department of Family Medicine, University of Washington, Seattle, WA 98195, USA;
[b] Department of Family Medicine, Family Medicine Residency of Idaho, 777 North Raymond Street, Boise, ID 83702, USA; [c] Department of Family Medicine, University of Washington School of Medicine, 331 North East Thornton Place, Seattle, WA 98125, USA
* Corresponding author. Family Medicine Residency of Idaho, Boise, ID 83704.
E-mail address: Danielle.davies@fmridaho.org

prolapse) or the full thickness of the wall of the rectum (complete prolapse).[1] The exact prevalence has not been well-characterized, but a small study estimated the incidence to be approximately 2.5 per 100,000 people annually with women being 9 times more likely to be affected.[2] Rectal prolapse can also be seen in children, most commonly in infancy. Rectal prolapse more commonly occurs in patients who are younger than 4 years of age than in those who are older.[3]

The exact cause of rectal prolapse has not been completely delineated. Risks factors seem to include constipation, multiparity, and pelvic floor dysfunction, among others.[1] Underlying conditions that are often associated with rectal prolapse in children include constipation, weakened pelvic floor muscles, and increased intraabdominal pressure. Additional consideration should be given to the presence of infectious diarrhea, diseases of the rectum including parasites and neoplasia, malnutrition, and cystic fibrosis.[2]

Because the process of rectal prolapse typically develops over time, affected adults often present complaining of a rectal bulge with defecation. Patients might also complain of fecal incontinence, bleeding, and pain. Diagnosis in the office setting usually involves reproducing the prolapse by having the patient perform the Valsalva maneuver in a squatting position or while on a commode. Partial prolapse involves just the rectal mucosa and is usually less pronounced than a complete prolapse, which involves the full thickness of the rectal wall. A complete prolapse typically involves a thick, fully circumferential red-colored prolapse demonstrating mucosal folds in circumferential rings. The orientation of the rectal mucosa folds in a partial prolapse run linearly from proximal to distal on the long axis of the intestine.[1] Rectal procidentia is described by grade in the case of a full-thickness prolapse and by degree in the case of mucosal prolapse (**Tables 1** and **2**).

If prolapse cannot be reproduced upon evaluation but is suspected by the history, defecography can be useful in making a diagnosis but cannot completely rule out prolapse.[4] Defecography, also referred to as evacuation or voiding proctography, involves the use of a barium paste inserted into the rectum followed by fluoroscopy or MRI while the patient passes the paste while sitting on a commode.[5] In children, the condition is often noticed by family members and has typically spontaneously reduced at the time of presentation. The diagnosis is inferred through the history.[3]

Rectal prolapse may or may not present with incarceration. Incarcerated rectal prolapses should have manual reduction attempted. Irreducibility is rare. Reduction is performed by encircling the prolapsed bowel with the fingertips and applying steady pressure, which may need to be quite firm if there is edema. Successful reduction should be followed by digital rectal examination.[3] If unsuccessful, subsequent attempts at reducing the prolapse can include use of local or general anesthesia to achieve relaxation of the pelvic floor musculature. Cold compresses can be applied to reduce swelling. In a case study of 15 patients with initially irreducible rectal procidentia, 4 patients had successful replacement with diclofenac or tramadol for pain relief, and 2 were successfully replaced after the application of simple table sugar

Table 1 Degree of partial rectal prolapse	
Degree	**Level of Mucosal Prolapse**
First	Into anal canal
Second	To dentate line
Third	To anal verge

Table 2
Grade of complete rectal prolapse

Grade	Level of Rectal Prolapse
I	Does not extend to level of rectocele
II	Does not extend to sphincter
III	Impinges on sphincter
IV	Enters the sphincter
V	Passes the sphincter

(an osmotic agent to reduce edema); 8 required general anesthesia. Five cases that included the application of sugar were not reduced successfully.[6] Overall there are few risks to the application of sugar. A prolapse that is not reduced may become necrotic or gangrenous, at which point surgical intervention will be required.[7] Cases of immediate recurrence of the prolapse can be treated by firmly affixing the buttocks together with tape for several hours.[3] Successfully reduced rectal prolapse can be treated with conservative medical management, which should aim at eliminating straining with bowel movements and increasing pelvic floor strength. Treatment of constipation is crucial. Medications aimed at creating soft bowel movements to minimize straining with defecation are listed in **Table 3**. No one medication is considered superior to another. It is this author's approach to use stool softeners and osmotic agents before prescribing bowel stimulants. In the case of a prolapse that is unable to be reduced manually, immediate referral to a surgeon should be made. Surgical consultation can also be made on an outpatient basis for those with recurrent prolapse (**see Table 3**)

ANAL FISSURE

Anal fissure has been estimated to have an annual incidence of 0.11% affecting approximately 1 person in 1000 yearly but study estimates varies widely. One retrospective population-based study found that the disorder more commonly affected females ages 12 to 24 and males 55 to 64 years of age.[8] Risk factors included chronic constipation, obesity, hypothyroidism, and solid tumors.[8]

Anal fissures are thought to be caused by the local trauma induced by inspissated feces. Anal spasm can additionally cause ischemia of sensitive rectal tissue, which exacerbates the condition.[9] The blood flow to the most common site of anal fissures is thought to be about one-half of that to other areas of the anal canal, creating an area of poor healing.[10]

Patients often complain of severe rectal pain, especially with bowel movements, described as sharp, "like passing shards of glass." Passage of blood is also possible, but is less common as the first presenting symptom. External examination can confirm the diagnosis. A small tear in the skin of the anus is present, most often in the posterior midline and begins at the dentate line and ends at the anal verge.[8] Fissures are classified into acute and chronic based on the duration of symptoms, acute meaning that symptoms have been present less than 2 to 3 months and chronic being defined as present for more than 3 months.[10]

Treatment is aimed at reducing anal spasm. Studies have compared the efficacy of watchful waiting, topical therapies (nifedipine, diltiazem, and nitroglycerin), internal sphincterotomy, and injection of botulinum toxin. A large Cochrane review, which compared the efficacy of 17 different therapies, established that topical nitroglycerin is better than placebo for anal fissures and is equivalent to botulinum toxin injection and topical calcium channel blockers. However, nitroglycerin tends to cause more

Table 3
Available therapies for constipation (cost estimated from Amazon.com and Goodrx.com)

Medication	Brand Names	Mechanism	Suggested Dose	Cost/Availability
Docusate sodium	Colace	Stool softener	100 mg BID	$5 for 400/OTC
Docusate calcium	Surfak	Stool softener	240 mg/d	$10/100/OTC
Polyethylene glycol	Miralax	Osmotic agent	17 g QD–BID	$10–13/510 g/OTC
Magnesium citrate	N/A	Osmotic agent	75–150 mL BID	$10/10oz/OTC
Lactulose	Kristalose	Osmotic agent	15–30 mL BID	$80/900 mL/prescription
Bisacodyl	Dulcolax Pink	Stimulant	5–15 mg QD	$5/1000 5 mg tab/OTC
Senna	Senokot	Stimulant	8.6 mg tablets up to 4 daily	$13/1000 8.6 mg tab/OTC
Psyllium	Metamucil	Bulk-forming agent	3.4 g up to TID	$25/1300 g/OTC
Methylcellulose	Citrucel	Bulk-forming agent	1 Tbsp up to TID	$12/454 g/OTC
Polycarbophil	FiberCon	Bulk-forming agent	2 tabs QD-QID	$20/140 tabs/OTC
Wheat dextrin	Benefiber	Bulk-forming agent	2 tsp TID	$20/25.6 oz/OTC

Abbreviations: BID, 2 times per day; OTC, over the counter; QD, once per day; QID, 4 times per day; TID, 3 times per day.

side effects, specifically headache. In the case of chronic fissures, surgical intervention is significantly more effective than medical management, but carries the additional risk of incontinence[11] Ongoing care aimed at reducing recurrence should focus on eliminating straining with bowel movements (**Table 4**).

Table 4
Therapies for anal fissure

Intervention	Studied Dosages	Effectiveness
NTG paste	0.2%–0.5% PR BID-TID for 4–8 weeks (all doses equal in effectiveness).	NNT = 7 for healing vs placebo, may have a higher recurrence rate vs surgery (up to 50% in medication use; headache most common side effect).[11]
Lidocaine	5% PR BID for 8 weeks.	Similar to NTG.[11]
Nifedipine	0.2%–0.3% BID for 3 weeks.	Similar to NTG.[11]
Botulinum toxin	20–50 IU injection, up to twice; superior healing rates were seen with anterior placement of Botox away from fissured area.	Similar to NTG. Effectiveness varied widely based on study design (40%–90% healing rates). No better or worse than NTG in head to head trials, NNT = 3 on placebo studies. Upwards of 50% recurrence rate at 1 year (transient mild incontinence presenting as main side effect in 7% of patients) seen most seen in.[11,33]
Diltiazem	2% topical. May also be used orally.	Similar to NTG.[11]
Clove oil	1% TID for 6 weeks.	Small studies; difficult to draw conclusions.[11]
Sitz bath	BID for 4 weeks.	May reduce anal pressure and burning with warm Sitz baths. No data found on cure rates, usually combined with medication.[11]
Sildenafil	10% TID for 7 days.	Relaxes anal tone. More studies needed to show if this could be of benefit.[11]
Isosorbide mononitrate	0.1% BID for 6 weeks.	Not as effective as topical preparations. May not be more effective than placebo.[11]
Isosorbide dinitrate	1% five time daily for 10 weeks.	Not as effective as topical preparations. May not be more effective than placebo.[11]
Sphincterotomy	Surgical cutting the anal sphincter.	There are 89% cure rates; 10% rate of anal incontinence (similar to Botox). Recurrence rate 3%.[11]

Abbreviations: BID, 2 times per day; NNT, number needed to treat; NTG, nitroglycerin; PR, per rectum; TID, 3 times per day.

HEMORRHOIDS

Hemorrhoids are one of the most common anorectal disorders to present to primary care offices. Because not all hemorrhoids cause symptoms, determining the exact prevalence has proven difficult. In the United States, a national survey showed that 4.4% of people complained of hemorrhoids.[12] Another study reported a finding of hemorrhoids in 39% of people presenting for routine colonoscopy with just under one-half of them reporting related symptoms.[13]

Increased intraabdominal pressure, as seen in chronic constipation, causes engorgement of the vascular plexuses surrounding the anal canal resulting in the development of hemorrhoids.[1] When this occurs above the dentate line, the superior hemorrhoidal plexus creates painless internal hemorrhoids. Conversely the inferior hemorrhoidal plexus gives rise to external hemorrhoids which are painful owing to their somatic innervation.[10]

Internal and external hemorrhoids are 2 very distinct entities when it comes to diagnosis, classification, and acute management. Internal hemorrhoids are classified based on a grading system. Grade 1 hemorrhoids do not extend distal to the dentate line. Grade 2 hemorrhoids may prolapse past the dentate line with straining but spontaneously reduce. Grade 3 hemorrhoids require manual reduction. Grade 4 hemorrhoids cannot be reduced manually[10] (**Table 5**).

External hemorrhoids do not have a similar grading system, but are classified as thrombosed versus nonthrombosed. The typical presenting complaints for external nonthrombosed hemorrhoids include itching and bleeding. In the case of thrombosed hemorrhoids, symptoms include bleeding, pain, and constipation.[14] Hemorrhoids are easily diagnosed on external rectal examination. External hemorrhoids also appear pink, but may become purple–blue when they become thrombosed and are usually quite tender.[15]

Internal hemorrhoids usually present with painless rectal bleeding. Grade 4 internal hemorrhoids may present with perineal irritation or pruritus, a sense of incomplete evacuation, or rectal fullness. When a prolapsed internal hemorrhoid becomes strangulated, patients most commonly complain of pain. Physical examination should ensure there is not a comorbid diagnosis such as anal fissure.[16] Careful physical examination including a digital rectal examination and anoscopy can diagnose internal hemorrhoids. They are typically purple–blue in appearance. Like external hemorrhoids, prolapsed internal hemorrhoids can be diagnosed by external examination of the anus. Prolapsed internal hemorrhoids typically appear as shiny pink protrusions. Although typically painless, a prolapsed internal hemorrhoid may be tender on palpation.[15]

Management of hemorrhoids depends their location, grade, and if thrombosis has occurred. In general, education and interventions should be aimed at therapies that avoid exacerbation of hemorrhoids along with symptomatic management. Avoiding

Table 5 Grades of internal hemorrhoids	
Grade	Definition
1	Enter lumen of bowel but do not extend to the dentate line.
2	Prolapse past the dentate line with straining but reduce with relaxation.
3	Prolapse past the dentate line with straining and require manual reduction.
4	Unable to be reduced.

exposure to prolonged periods of increased rectal pressure can help to prevent the formation of both internal and external hemorrhoids. Therapies in this case should focus on creating soft bowel movements through the use of fiber supplements or other bulk-forming agents (see **Table 3**). Fiber therapy alone was found to reduce overall symptoms by 53% (relative risk, 0.47; 95% CI, 0.32–0.68).[17] Patients should also be educated in avoiding prolonged periods of time on the toilet.[15] About one-half of patients will have improvement of internal hemorrhoids with conservative therapy.

For grades 1 to 3 internal hemorrhoids, rubber band ligation, sclerotherapy, and infrared coagulation can be used in the primary care office. There remains some controversy about the most effective strategy for in-office treatment. Two large meta-analyses showed that those treated with rubber band ligation were more likely to have resolution of hemorrhoids at the 1-year follow-up, although patients experienced more postoperative pain.[18,19] There are a variety of commercially available rubber band ligators that can be used in the primary care office. Traditionally, in conjunction with an anoscope, the instrument uses suction to draw the hemorrhoid into the instrument and a rubber band is deployed around the base of the hemorrhoid.[16] Sclerotherapy uses caustic agents injected at the base of grades 1 to 3 hemorrhoids and is effective in 75% to 89% of cases. Although sclerotherapeutic preparations may vary, 1 mL of 10% phenol can be injected using a 21- or 25-gauge spinal needle into the base of the hemorrhoid under direct visualization.[20] Infrared coagulation (a concentrated light that is used to produce a predictable shallow burn that causes the layers of the hemorrhoid vessel to scar to each other) also can achieve sclerosis of the hemorrhoidal tissue and has been shown to be less painful in studies.[20] Hemorrhoids are treated with 1.5 seconds of exposure with 3 subsequent burns placed in a row or diamond pattern above the hemorrhoid being treated.[20] No more than 2 separate hemorrhoids should be treated per session. Surgical management, such as excisional hemorrhoidectomy and stapled hemorrhoidopexy, should be reserved for persistent grade 3 hemorrhoids and grade 4 internal hemorrhoids because, although effective, there are increased side effects associated with surgical management, most notably postoperative pain.[14] Further consideration is not given here to surgical approaches including Doppler-guided transanal ligation, owing to their lack of applicability in the primary care office setting.

External hemorrhoids can be managed with topical preparations, most of which are available over the counter. Sitz baths can help with edema of external hemorrhoids and internal prolapsed hemorrhoids. Topical corticosteroids can be effective in decreasing irritation associated with hemorrhoids but should not be used for greater than a week owing to the risk of skin atrophy. Topical therapy with mineral oil, petrolatum, and phenylephrine can provide relief, although these products do not treat hemorrhoids or prevent progression or recurrence. A topical preparation of nifedipine and lidocaine ointment can be compounded and may help with resolution of acutely thrombosed external hemorrhoids and alleviation of pain. A small study of 98 patients compared topical 0.3% nifedipine with 1.5% lidocaine twice daily for 12 weeks with a control group using topical lidocaine alone. Symptomatic relief was obtained within 7 days of therapy in 86% of patients versus 50% in the control group ($P <.01$). Resolution of the thrombosis at the 2-week mark occurred in 92% of patients in the treatment group versus 46% in the control group.[21] Thrombosed external hemorrhoids presenting within 72 hours of symptom onset can be evacuated in the clinic.[1] Beyond 72 hours, studies have shown increased postprocedure pain after evacuation. Consideration should be given to surgical intervention when patients have worsening rather than improving pain. Thrombosed external hemorrhoids may be removed in the office setting by first injecting the area with a local anesthetic. An elliptical incision is made over the hemorrhoid, excising the entire thrombus rather than simply lancing out part of the clot. Patients can be instructed to use Sitz baths at home and over-the-counter preparations for continued wound care at home.[20]

PROCTALGIA FUGAX

Proctalgia fugax is a disorder characterized by sharp pain that passes quickly in the rectum. Prevalence rates are as high as 18% in the general population. Onset is unlikely before puberty.[22]

The pathophysiology of proctalgia fugax is not fully understood and may result from smooth muscle contractions.[23] Several studies have tried to measure intraluminal pressures in the anorectal vicinity during an episode. Findings in these studies were inconsistent. One study demonstrated increased sigmoid pressure during an attack.[22] Another found increased baseline resting pressures with increased anal sphincter tone, and slow wave smooth muscle activity during an attack.[22] There has reportedly been an association with intercourse, masturbation, stress, defecation, sitting in a chair, drinking alcohol, cold nights, sexual frustration, and menstruation, but episodes can also occur spontaneously. Historically speaking, proctalgia fugax has been associated with neuroticism, perfectionism, and anxiety, and some studies supported this finding, although only correlation, not causation, has been established.[22]

Proctalgia fugax may be diagnosed when the patient reports recurrent episodes of rectal pain, lasting less than 30 minutes. These episodes are not associated with defecation and patients do not experience pain between episodes. Other causes of rectal pain must be excluded, including inflammatory bowel disease, rectal abscess, rectal fissure, thrombosed hemorrhoid, prostatitis, coccygodynia, and major structural alterations of the pelvic floor such as pelvic organ prolapse.[22] However, the presence of another diagnosis does not exclude patients from also having proctalgia fugax. Fifty percent of patients will have up to 5 attacks yearly.[23]

Often, attacks of proctalgia fugax are self-limited and brief, making treatment unnecessary. Numerous treatment modalities have been tried and aim to induce sphincter relaxation. Suggested interventions include anorectal digital dilation, activation of the anorectal reflex through food consumption, position changes including knees to chest, hot baths, and forced evacuation of the rectum. In case reports, topical 2% diltiazem and 0.2% glyceryl trinitrate have been effective. Oral calcium channel blockers, clonidine, and intravenous lidocaine have also been effective in case reports, but no trials have proved significant efficacy.[22] For patients with longer lasting episodes (>20 minutes), a small study did show some evidence that inhaled salbutamol shortened the duration and severity of attacks compared with placebo.[24] A small trial of 5 patients with proctalgia fugax were treated with 25 IU of botulinum A toxin. Only 1 patient required a supplementary dose of 50 IU and all patients remained symptom free at the 2-year point.[25] In some cases, endoanal ultrasound examination has identified a thickened internal anal sphincter, and 1 case report suggested that this was familial. Limited internal anal sphincterotomy has been effective in these cases.[22] Therapy should aim at reassurance. Conservative treatment measures are usually indicated owing to the fleeting nature of symptoms. For those patients with persistent bothersome symptoms an algorithm (**Fig. 1**) can be used for escalating therapy.

LEVATOR ANI SYNDROME

Levator ani syndrome, also known as levator spasm, puborectalis syndrome, chronic proctalgia, pyriformis syndrome, and pelvic tension myalgia, affects approximately

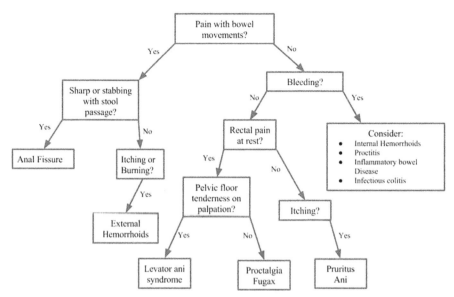

Fig. 1. Algorithm to aid in the approach to diagnosis of common anorectal disorders.

6.6% of the population with an estimated one-third of affected individuals seeking medical attention for symptomatic relief.[26] To meet the criteria for diagnosis of levator ani syndrome, patients must have chronic or recurrent rectal pain or aching with episodes lasting for longer than 30 minutes and tenderness during posterior traction of the puborectalis muscle. There can be no other causes of pain, including inflammatory bowel disease, rectal abscess, rectal fissure, thrombosed hemorrhoid, or major structural alterations of the pelvic floor (such as pelvic organ prolapse or prior surgical intervention). These criteria must be fulfilled for the previous 3 months with onset at least 6 months prior.[23]

Patients usually complain of a dull aching sensation in the rectum. Provoking factors may include sitting and patients may report improvement with laying down or standing. Digital rectal examination should be undertaken in the office. The examiner may note increased tone in the levator ani muscles and tenderness of the pelvic floor, which is often worse on the left. Because the diagnostic criteria require ruling out several other differential diagnoses, patient with suspected levator ani syndrome will likely need further workup with appropriate testing.[26]

Therapies are limited and treatment is typically challenging, especially because patients may have comorbid psychiatric illness and/or neurotic tendencies. A prospective, randomized, controlled trial compared the effectiveness of biofeedback focusing on pelvic floor relaxation, electrogalvanic stimulation, and levator muscle ,massage and found that patients in the biofeedback group had the greatest reduction in intensity and frequency of pain symptoms.[27] A small study did not show any improvement with botulinum toxin injection into the levator muscles.[28]

PRURITUS ANI

Pruritis ani is described as an intense itch affecting the perianal area. Because many patients do not present to care, the epidemiology is difficult to obtain but it is estimated that 1% to 5% of the population suffers from perianal itching.[14]

There are a multitude of primary inciting causes of pruritus ani. The general cycle includes an initial irritative event causing pruritus, which incites scratching by the patient and intensification of the pruritus.[14] More than 100 different inciting events have described, and a complete listing is not included here. Contact dermatitis, certain foods, hemorrhoids, dermatologic conditions, hygiene issues including fecal soiling, medications, soaps, and clothing are among some of the commonly described inciting factors.[29]

Patients who present with anal itching should undergo rectal examination to check for treatable causative agent, including pinworms and hemorrhoids. Because dermatologic conditions can exist that cause perianal itching, skin distant to the anus should also be examined. In chronic pruritus ani, examination of the anus may reveal lichenification (often identified as fine white linear markings on the thickened skin).[30] Pruritus ani can either exist by itself or in combination with its inciting event. Examination should focus on identifying other treatable conditions that may be exacerbating symptoms.

Treatment should focus on stopping the itch–scratch cycle and maintaining proper hygiene. The first step should be avoiding inciting events. Patients should be advised to avoid irritants such as soaps, bubble baths cleansers, and certain foods (caffeinated beverages, alcohol, chocolate, tomatoes, spicy foods, prunes, figs, milk, spices, citrus, grapes, popcorn, and nuts). Because both a lack of hygiene and aggressive cleaning can initiate the cycle, gentle cleansing of the anus after bowel movements should be stressed. A barrier cream can be applied as well.[29] Because many patients may unknowingly contribute to the scratch–itch cycle while sleeping, medications that reduce itching including diphenhydramine and hydroxyzine can be given before sleep to aid in the reduction of scratching at night.[14] Medications are available for refractory cases. Topical 0.006% capsaicin was shown to be more effective than a menthol placebo in controlling pruritus in a small study.[31] Another study demonstrated efficacy of 1% hydrocortisone ointment as compared with placebo.[32] Anal tattooing with methylene blue is available for the most refractory cases. Subcutaneous and intradermal injections of 10 mL 1% methylene blue, 5 mL normal saline, 7.5 mL 0.25% bupivacaine with epinephrine, and 7.5 mL 0.5% lignocaine may help a small subset of patients, but does carry the risk of skin necrosis.[29] In summary, treatment should focus on eliminating inciting factors, treating the chronic pruritis, and educating the patient about the disease course.

REFERENCES

1. Fox A, Tietze PH, Ramakrishnan K. Anorectal conditions. FP Essentials™. Edition No. 419. Leawood (KS): American Academy of Family Physicians; 2014.

2. Kairaluoma MV, Kellokumpu IH. Epidemiologic aspects of complete rectal prolapse. Scand J Surg 2005;94(3):207–10.

3. Siafakas C, Vottler TP, Andersen JM. Rectal prolapse in pediatrics. Clin Pediatr (Phila) 1999;38(2):63–72.

4. Mellgren A, Bremmer S, Johansson C, et al. Defecography. Results of investigations in 2,816 patients. Dis Colon Rectum 1994;37:1133–41.

5. Kim AY. How to interpret a functional or motility test - defecography. J Neurogastroenterol Motil 2011;17(4):416–20.

6. Seenivasagam T, Gerald H, Ghassan N, et al. Irreducible rectal prolapse: emergency surgical management of eight cases and a review of the literature. Med J Malaysia 2011;66(2):105–7.

7. Goldstein SD, Maxwell PJ. Rectal prolapse. Clin Colon Rectal Surg 2011;24(1): 39–45.
8. Mapel DW, Schum M, Von Worley A. The epidemiology and treatment of anal fissures in a population-based cohort. BMC Gastroenterol 2014;14:129.
9. Wray D, Ijaz S, Lidder S. Anal fissure: a review. Br J Hosp Med (Lond) 2008;69(8): 455–8.
10. Foxx-Orenstein AE, Umar SB, Crowell MD. Common anorectal disorders. Gastroenterol Hepatol 2014;10(5):294–301.
11. Nelson RL, Thomas K, Morgan J, et al. Non surgical therapy for anal fissure. Cochrane Database Syst Rev 2012;(2):CD003431.
12. Johanson JF, Sonnenberg A. The prevalence of hemorrhoids and chronic constipation. An epidemiologic study. Gastroenterology 1990;98(2):380–6.
13. Riss S, Weiser FA, Schwameis K, et al. The prevalence of hemorrhoids in adults. Int J Colorectal Dis 2011;27(2):215–20.
14. Fargo MV, Latimer KM. Evaluation and management of common anorectal conditions. Am Fam Physician 2012;85(6):624–30.
15. Mounsey AL, Halladay J, Sadiq TS. Hemorrhoids. Am Fam Physician 2011;84(2): 204–10.
16. Lohsiriwat V. Hemorrhoids: from basic pathophysiology to clinical management. World J Gastroenterol 2012;18(17):2009–17.
17. Alonso-coello P, Mills E, Heels-ansdell D, et al. Fiber for the treatment of hemorrhoids complications: a systematic review and meta-analysis. Am J Gastroenterol 2006;101(1):181–8.
18. Johanson JF, Rimm A. Optimal nonsurgical treatment of hemorrhoids: a comparative analysis of infrared coagulation, rubber band ligation, and injection sclerotherapy. Am J Gastroenterol 1992;87(11):1600–6.
19. MacRae HM, McLeod RS. Comparison of hemorrhoidal treatments: a meta-analysis. Can J Surg 1997;40(1):14–7.
20. Sanchez C, Chinn BT. Hemorrhoids. Clin Colon Rectal Surg 2011;24(1):5–13.
21. Perrotti P, Antopoli C, Molino D, et al. Conservative treatment of acute thrombosed external hemorrhoids with topical nifedipine. Dis Colon Rectum 2001;44: 405–9.
22. Jeyarajah S, Chow A, Ziprin P, et al. Proctalgia fugax, an evidence-based management pathway. Int J Colorectal Dis 2010;25:1037–46.
23. Rao SS, Bharucha AE, Chiarioni G, et al. Functional anorectal disorders. Gastroenterology 2016;150(6):1430–42.
24. Eckardt VF, Dodt O, Kanzler G, et al. Treatment of proctalgia fugax with salbutamol inhalation. Am J Gastroenterol 1996;91(4):686–9.
25. Sánchez romero AM, Arroyo sebastián A, Pérez vicente FA, et al. Treatment of proctalgia fugax with botulinum toxin: results in 5 patients. Rev Clin Esp 2006; 206(3):137–40.
26. Bharucha AE, Wald AM. Anorectal disorders. Am J Gastroenterol 2010;105(4): 786–94.
27. Chiarioni G, Nardo A, Vantini I, et al. Biofeedback is superior to electrogalvanic stimulation and massage for treatment of levator ani syndrome. Gastroenterology 2010;138(4):1321–9.
28. Rao SS, Paulson J, Mata M, et al. Clinical trial: effects of botulinum toxin on levator ani syndrome: a double blind, placebo controlled study. Aliment Pharmacol Ther 2009;29(9):985–91.
29. Siddiqi S, Vijay V, Ward M, et al. Pruritus ani. Ann R Coll Surg Engl 2008;90(6): 457–63.

30. Pfenninger JL, Zainea GG. Common anorectal conditions: part I. Symptoms and complaints. Am Fam Physician 2001;63(12):2391–8.
31. Lysy J, Sistiery-Ittah M, Israelit Y, et al. Topical capsaicin—a novel and effective treatment for idiopathic intractable pruritus ani: a randomised, placebo controlled, crossover study. Gut 2003;52(9):1323–6.
32. Al-ghnaniem R, Short K, Pullen A, et al. 1% hydrocortisone ointment is an effective treatment of pruritus ani: a pilot randomized controlled crossover trial. Int J Colorectal Dis 2007;22(12):1463–7.
33. Brisinda G, Cadeddu F, Brandara F, et al. Randomized clinical trial comparing botulinum toxin injections with 0.2 per cent nitroglycerin ointment for chronic anal fissure. Br J Surg 2007;94(2):162–7.

Gastrointestinal Malignancies

William R. Sonnenberg, MD, FAAPF[a,b],*

KEYWORDS

- Esophageal • Cancer • Malignancy • Gastric • Colon • Helicobacter • Pylori

KEY POINTS

- Esophageal cancer is one of the few cancers that is increasing in incidence in the United States. Symptoms are nonspecific and present late.
- Preventive measures include weight control, increasing consumption of fruits and vegetables, smoking cessation, alcohol limitation, and fiber.
- Gastric cancer has been on the decline for decades, largely owing to improved sanitation and treatment of *Helicobacter pylori* infection.
- There are no screening recommendations in the United States for gastric cancer.
- Colon cancer is the third most common cancer and the second leading cause of death in the United States. Screening is effective and has the potential of reducing death by 50%.

INTRODUCTION

This article discusses 3 gastrointestinal malignancies: esophageal, gastric, and colorectal. Anne Walling and Robert Freelove's article "Pancreatitis and Pancreatic Cancer," elsewhere in this issue. Collectively, these 3 cancers are responsible for 22% of cancer deaths in the United States. It is estimated that 90% of all cancers in the United States are the result of environmental exposures, and the gastrointestinal malignancies certainly are associated with those exposures. These outside insults include dietary intake, tobacco use, alcohol consumption, obesity, and pathogens. Osler said of the stomach, "The stomach is the hardest worked and most abused organ of the body, more subject also to irritation than any other." It is certain that Osler would also agree that the esophagus and colon are victims of these same irritants (**Table 1**).

ESOPHAGEAL CANCER

Perhaps one of the most distressing cancer diagnosis for both the patient and the physician is esophageal cancer (**Fig. 1**). It is estimated in 2016 there will be 16,910

Disclosure Statement: The author has nothing to disclose.
[a] Titusville Area Hospital, 406 West Spruce Street, Titusville, PA 16354, USA; [b] Department of Family & Community Medicine, Penn State Milton S. Hershey Medical Center, 500 University Dr., H154/C1626, Hershey, PA 17033, USA
* Corresponding author. 119 East Mechanic Street, Titusville, PA 16354.
E-mail address: drbill@drbillfp.com

Table 1
Incidence and deaths of gastrointestinal cancer by sites in the United States, 2013

Site	Incidence	Deaths
Colorectal	142,820	50,830
Pancreas	45,220	38,460
Gastric	21,660	10,990
Esophagus	17,990	15,210

Data from Siegel R, Naishadham D, Jemal A. Cancer statistics, 2013. CA Cancer J Clin 2013;63:12.

new cases and 15,690 deaths per year. The mean age at diagnosis is 67 and mean age of death is 69. It is more common in men at a ratio of 3 to 4:1. It is the 11th leading cause of cancer death, yet ranks as the 18th most common cancer. The lifetime risk of getting esophageal cancer is 0.5%.[1]

Ninety-five percent of esophageal cancers are epithelial in origin and there are 2 main types, squamous cell and adenocarcinoma.[2] Squamous cell carcinoma is the predominant esophageal cancer in the developing world and responsible for 90% of cancers worldwide. Risk factors for squamous cell esophageal cancer seem to be associated with lifestyle factors, such as smoking tobacco and alcohol consumption. Consumption of 3 or more drinks per day increases this risk 3 to 5 times.[3] It seems that beer and spirits carry the highest risk. Those who heavily smoke black tobacco and drink alcohol may be cursed with an odds ratio for developing esophageal cancer of greater than 100-fold.[4] Other risk factors include being male or black, having had thoracic radiation therapy or a history of lye ingestion, and consuming a high-starch diet lacking in fruits and vegetables.[5]

Adenocarcinoma is more of a cancer of the developed world and is replacing squamous cell carcinoma as the most common cancer in the United States and Western Europe.[6] Currently in the United States, it accounts for 70% of esophageal cancers. The incidence is increasing faster than any other cancer in the United States.[7] Unlike squamous cell carcinoma, adenocarcinoma is less associated with alcohol consumption. Current smokers have twice the risk as nonsmokers of developing adenocarcinoma of the esophagus, but smoking is still less of an etiologic factor than it is for

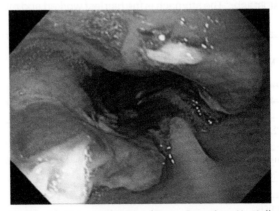

Fig. 1. Adenocarcinoma of the esophagus. (*From* Banerjee N, Adler DG. Malignant dysphagia: evaluation and endoscopic treatment. In: Davis MP, Feyer PC, Ortner P, et al, editors. Supportive oncology. Chapter 17. Saunders; 2011. p. 172; with permission.)

squamous cell esophageal cancer.[8] The stronger risk factors for adenocarcinoma are obesity and gastroesophageal reflux disease (GERD). Persons with weekly symptoms of GERD have 5 times the risk and those with daily GERD symptoms have a 7-fold increase in risk.[3] Obesity increases the risk 2.4 to 2.8 times.[9] Abdominal obesity is associated with Barrett esophagus and cancer. Because men have more abdominal adiposity, this has been postulated as the reason more men than women develop esophageal cancer.

Certain factors have been shown to reduce the risk of esophageal cancer. One of the more provocative and interesting is the protective effect of infection with Helicobacter pylori. Despite being a known risk factor for gastric cancer, H pylori–infected populations have been shown by metaanalysis to have a 41% decreased risk of adenocarcinoma of esophagus.[10] It is felt that gastric atrophy caused by H pylori leads to less acid production and less Barrett esophagus. Esophageal squamous cell carcinoma seems unaffected by H pylori.[11] High intake of fiber, fresh fruit, and vegetables lowers the risk of both cancers (**Table 2**).

Symptoms of esophageal cancer tend to be vague for 2 to 4 months before coming to medical attention. Typical symptoms usually do not occur until the tumor has infiltrated the lumen to more than 60% of the circumference.[12] At that point, the cancer is in advanced stages. The first typical symptom is usually difficulty in swallowing dry foods or breads. Later there are problems with liquids. They may have had an unexplained weight loss, which occurs 50% of the time. Later symptoms include pain on swallowing, halitosis, hoarseness, or hiccups. Another common presentation is heartburn unresponsive to medical treatment. Hoarseness is caused by invasion of the recurrent laryngeal nerve; at this stage, the disease cannot be resected surgically. An intractable cough and recurrent pneumonia may develop owing to recurrent aspiration or a tracheobronchial fistula.

Physical examination is of little help. Signs of weight loss may be present. Lymphadenopathy may be noted in the laterocervical or supraclavicular nodes. There may be hepatomegaly.

Screening for adenocarcinoma is directed at Barrett esophagus, a precursor of esophageal adenocarcinoma where columnar epithelium replaces normal squamous epithelium. The annual risk for cancer with nondysplastic Barrett esophagus is 0.12% to 0.40%[13] Barrett esophagus with dysplasia has a much higher risk; 1% for low-grade dysplasia and 5% annual risk for high-grade dysplasia. Of the patients with prolonged GERD symptoms, 6% to 12% have Barrett esophagus. White males

Table 2	
Esophageal cancer risk factors	
Squamous Cell	**Adenocarcinoma**
Tobacco	Symptomatic gastroesophageal reflux disease
Alcohol	Barrett esophagus
Enzyme mutations for alcohol metabolism	Obesity
Achalasia	Tobacco
Thoracic radiation	Thoracic radiation
Low socioeconomic status	Diet low in fruits and vegetables
Poor oral hygiene	Age
Nutritional deficiencies	Male sex

Adapted from Pennathur A, Gibson MK, Jobe BA, et al. Oesophageal carcinoma. Lancet 2013;381(9864):401; with permission.

older than 50 years of age are the most likely to have Barrett esophagus.[13] The impression from observational studies shows that patients undergoing surveillance tend to have early stage cancer, and may have prolonged survival.

Complimenting endoscopic surveillance is radiofrequency ablation of low- or high-grade Barrett esophagus. The procedure results in resolution of esophageal metaplasia in 77% of cases and 86% of dysplasia.[14] This results in a lower risk of progression and fewer cancers. Regular, long-term follow-up shows that the benefit is durable. Recurrences occur, but they are usually nondysplastic and readily handled endoscopically.

Preventing esophageal cancer should start with the classic recommendations common to many diseases. Tobacco cessation, moderation of alcohol use, maintenance of ideal body weight, and consuming a diet high in fruits and vegetables should be advocated. The National Cancer Institute notes that, "diets high in cruciferous (cabbage, broccoli/broccolini, cauliflower, Brussels sprouts) and green and yellow vegetables and fruits are associated with a decreased risk of esophageal cancer."[15] Dietary fiber is felt to decrease risk, especially of adenocarcinoma.[16]

Proton pump inhibitors have been significantly associated with a reduction in risk of high-grade dysplasia and adenocarcinoma in Barrett esophagus.[17] Oddly, several cohort studies have failed to show that antireflux surgery reduces the risk of adenocarcinoma in patients with GERD or Barrett esophagus.[9] Observational studies have shown a risk reduction of 40% to 50% with aspirin or nonsteroidal antiinflammatory drugs (NSAIDs). Other studies show that celecoxib shows no risk reduction in Barrett esophagus, dysplasia, or squamous dysplasia.[9]

It seems incredible that there seems to be no end to the diseases that statins reduce the risk, and adenocarcinoma of the esophagus can be added to this list. A metaanalysis of 13 studies showed that statin users have a 28% reduction of esophageal adenocarcinoma in and a 41% reduction of Barrett esophagus.[18]

GASTRIC CANCER

Gastric cancer is both an aggressive neoplasm and yet has been retreating in incidence over the past decades (**Fig. 2**). The incidence of the cancer is one of the most common worldwide, but is decreasing in the western world. Before the 1930s, gastric cancer was a leading cause of cancer death in the United States. It is now the 13th leading cause of death in this country,[19] but for the rest of the world, it is the third leading cause of death. Even as gastric cancer is decreasing, the location of the cancer is moving toward the gastroesophageal junction. This decrease may be linked to improved water supply, refrigeration of food, fewer infections, and improved dietary habits.[20] The same Western lifestyle that may be increasing adenocarcinoma of the esophagus may result in decreasing gastric cancer rates. The male/female ratio is 1.7:1 and the predominant age is older than 55 years.

Infection with H pylori is the primary risk factor for gastric cancer. This is the first time that a bacterium has been associated with any cancer. It is felt that 65% to 80% of gastric cancer is caused by H pylori, but only 2% of those infected get gastric cancer. H pylori causes chronic inflammation and cell proliferation, which increases the risk of DNA damage. Acquiring H pylori at an earlier age increases risk. The cagA strain is more toxigenic and is associated with a 2 to 3 times greater risk.[21] It remains unclear whether eradication of H pylori decreases the risk of cancer, although some studies are suggestive. One study, using pooled data from 5 studies in Asia showed the risk of gastric cancer was reduced almost in half with eradication of H pylori.[22] Epstein-Barr virus has been associated with some gastric cancers, but again the role is unclear (**Table 3**).

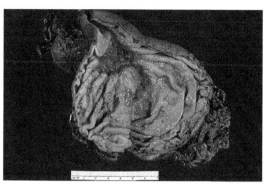

Fig. 2. Adenocarcinoma of the stomach. (*From* Keenan NG, Nicholson AG, Oldershawa PJ. Fatal acute pulmonary hypertension caused by pulmonary tumour thrombotic microangiop athy. Int J Cardiol 2008;124(1):e11–3; with permission.)

Other risk factors include tobacco use, a diet low in fruits and vegetables, and salted, smoked, or pickled foods. Obesity seldom helps with any risk factor, and gastric cancer is no exception. It is associated with a risk factor of 1.22.[29] Being obese and having GERD is clearly related to gastroesophageal junction cancers. Alcohol does not seem to be associated with gastric cancer.[30]

Probably 90% of gastric cancers are sporadic and environmental, but about 10% seem to involve familial clustering. Defined genetic syndromes are involved in 2% to 3%.[31] One syndrome is hereditary diffuse gastric cancer, which is autosomal domi-nant. It has high penetrance and high mortality. It occurs at a young age. Genetic testing can be done. Individuals at high risk should be monitored aggressively or un-dergo prophylactic gastrectomy.

Screening on a routine basis for the general population has not been found to be practical in the West. Countries such as Japan, with a higher risk of gastric cancer, have rigorous screening programs that identify gastric cancer early. Endoscopy is started at age 50. Screening in the United States should be considered in those with a known genetic predisposition.

Sadly, most gastric cancers cause symptoms only in the late stages, resulting in the diagnosis being made late in the disease process. Unintentional weight loss is the most common symptom, occurring in 70% to 80% of people who are diagnosed. Other common symptoms at presentation are anorexia, early satiety, dyspepsia, and abdominal pain. Tumors at the gastroesophageal junction present with dysphagia. These symptoms occur at a late stage.

Table 3	
Risk factors of gastric cancer	
Risk Factor	**Odds Ratio**
Helicobacter pylori infection	2.97[23]
High salt intake	1.68[24]
Fruit intake	0.82[25]
Vegetables	0.88
Western diet	1.51[26]
Green tea (only women)	0.70[27]
Smoking (30 cigarettes/d)	1.70[28]

Physical examination may show a palpably enlarged stomach, hepatomegaly, jaundice, or ascites. Metastatic lymphadenopathy may show up as a Virchow's node (left supraclavicular), Sister Mary Joseph's nodule (periumbilical), or a Blumer's shelf node (rectal).

In today's world, esophagogastroduodenoscopy is usually the first and preferred step in the workup. Six biopsies should be performed at a minimum.[32] Esophagogastroduodenoscopy has a 95% diagnostic accuracy. Double-contrast radiologic imaging can be done for cost savings and as a noninvasive option. Benign-appearing gastric ulcers can rule out gastric cancer 95% of the times. Overall, the upper gastrointestinal radiologic imaging has a diagnostic accuracy of 75%. Too often imaging is indeterminate and esophagogastroduodenoscopy must be performed for diagnostic certainty. Other tests include complete blood count, chemistry panel, H pylori testing, and computed tomography scans of the chest, abdomen, and pelvis with contrast and gastric distension for staging.

Histologically, 90% to 95% of gastric cancers are adenocarcinomas. The second most common is lymphoma. Leiomyomas or leiomyosarcomas account for 2%. Carcinoids, adenoacanthomas, and squamous cell carcinomas comprise the remaining histologic types. Prognosis depends on the depth of cancer invasion and regional lymph node involvement. The greater number of involved lymph nodes, the greater the chance of poor outcome after surgery. Postoperative margins that are positive for cancer are associated with a very poor prognosis.

Treatment of gastric cancer is complex, requiring a multidisciplinary team. Only 40% of patients in the West are candidates for potentially curative surgery. The type of surgery depends the location of the tumor, whether it is proximal or distal. The lymphatic network of the stomach is extensive; thus, a 5-cm margin of resection, both proximal and distal, should be attempted. The extent of lymph node dissection is controversial. More extensive dissection is recommended by the National Comprehensive Network.[33] Lesser dissections have fewer anastomotic leaks, lower postoperative complications, shorter duration of stay, and lower 30-day mortality. Survival at 5 years is similar.[34]

Radiation therapy often has a role. Targeted intraoperative radiation allows a high dose of radiation to be focused on diseased tissue in the operating room and avoids collateral damage to other structures. Survival seems to be improved (21 months vs 10 months), but is not statistically significant.[35] Postoperative adjunct radiation seems to help in both overall and relapse-free survival.

Because most patients with gastric cancer present in the advanced state, palliative treatment is the preferred management option. Distant metastases, carcinomatosis, unresectable liver metastases, pulmonary metastases, and direct local invasion may complicate the patient's course. Radiation therapy may help with the management of bleeding, obstruction, and pain. Surgical procedures may be required to allow food intake and lessen pain. A variety of chemotherapy agents have been tried and more studies are pending.

Overall, the prognosis for gastric cancer is poor. Only a small percentage of patients undergoing surgical resection will be cured. A reoperation trial at 6 months at the University of Minnesota showed that the local recurrence rate is 67%, gastric bed 54%, and regional nodes 42%; 26% of patients had distant failure.[36]

COLON CANCER

It is relatively gratifying to conclude this article with the topic of colon cancer. Screening is effective and treatment has a better chance of succeeding. Colon cancer is the third most common cancer in both males and females in the United States, and the second leading cause of cancer death in the United States.[37] Mortality increases after the age of 50 to the age of 80. It is estimated that full implementation of colon cancer screening guidelines could reduce colon cancer deaths by 50%[38] The highest incidence and mortality occurs in African American men and women.[39]

Mortality for colorectal cancer has decreased by 30% between 2000 and 2010 in both sexes and all races.[40] This improvement may be due to increased screening rates, earlier detection, and better treatment. Other factors may account for this improvement. The US population smokes less, use more aspirin for heart health, and uses more over-the-counter NSAIDs.

Risk factors for colon cancer are numerous, but often center around the usual suspects common to many cancers. A prospective study suggests obesity is a risk factor with the relative risk increasing with increasing body mass indexes to an relative risk of 1.84 at a body mass index of 35.0 to 39.9 kg/m^2.[41] Dietary fat seems to increase risk, possibly by increasing bile acid in the colon. The relative risk of a high-fat diet may be as high as 2.2.[42] Dietary fat has also been associated with more recurrences of adenomas after polypectomy. Red meat and a lack of fiber may increase risk, but the data lack consistency. Although it is difficult not to feel that a diet high in fruits and vegetables would lower the risk of colon cancer, studies have failed to endorse the benefit, including a large, prospective study.[43]

Regular physical activity provides a gratifying relative risk reduction of 40%[44] and lower mortality after colon resection surgery.[45] Smoking is also a modifiable risk factor; heavy smokers have a 2- to 3-fold greater risk of adenocarcinoma than nonsmokers. It is the possible that cigarettes may be associated with 1 in 5 colon cancers in the United States.[46]

The most common inherited genetic syndrome associated with colon cancer is Lynch syndrome, an autosomal-dominant disorder associated with up to 6% of colon cancers. It is associated with fewer polyps than hereditary familial polyposis. The genetic problem is a defect in DNA mismatch repair. The lifetime risk for colon cancer is 80% and the average age at diagnosis is 55 years. The risk is higher in men. Two-thirds of the cancers occur in the proximal colon. The only proven screening procedure is serial colonoscopies every 1 to 2 years starting at age 25.

Another genetic syndrome is familial adenomatous polyposis. It is characterized by thousands of small polyps less than 1 cm in diameter, throughout the entire large bowel. The polyps develop in the second or third decade of life. Cancer is a near certainty by age 40. Genetic testing, preceded by counseling, is the standard of care. There is a clear value in screening relatives of the affected family member.[47] A sigmoidoscopy should be performed at 10 to 12 years of age with mucosal biopsies. Full colonoscopy should begin at 18 to 20.

Two classes of medications seem to reduce the risk of colon cancer. Postmenopausal hormone therapy has shown a decreased risk in multiple studies. The famous Women's Health Initiative showed a benefit of estrogen and progesterone combination, reducing risk by 44%.[48] NSAIDs and aspirin have been associated with a reduced risk of colorectal adenomas, colorectal cancer, and colon cancer mortality. A large prospective study of 660,000 adults found a 40% reduction in rectal and colon cancer mortality in regular users of aspirin.[49]

Symptoms of colon cancer are microcytic anemia, rectal bleeding, pain, change in bowel habit, obstruction, or perforation. Lesions of the right-sided ascending colon are more likely to present as bleeding and diarrhea because the stool is more liquid. Lesions of the left colon are more likely to present as obstruction. Fortunately, because of increased screening, more cancers are being diagnosed before symptoms are apparent.

Unlike esophageal and gastric cancers, screening for colon cancer is established in the United States and it works. In contrast with screening programs for lung, prostate, and breast cancers, screening for colon cancer can detect precancerous lesions in addition to early cancer. A 2013 study involving almost 89,000 participants showed a hazard ratio of death from colon cancer of 0.59 for screening sigmoidoscopy and 0.32 for screening colonoscopy. Screening sigmoidoscopy does not reduce death from proximal colon cancer, which would be anticipated.[50] Another study involving more than 46,000 participants using fecal occult blood testing (FOBT) on an annual or biannual basis showed a relative risk of death from colon cancer of 0.68.[51] Screening has been shown to reduce the chance of dying from colon cancer from 40% to almost 70%. Screening is also cost effective. The estimated cost of 1 year of life gained with screening is $20,000 to $40,000.[52] In each year, only 10% of adults visiting a doctor received a colon screening recommendation.[53] Only 60% to 65% of those older than age 50 have undergone one of the recommended screening tests.[54]

Most guidelines suggest beginning screening in average risk patients at age 50. The American College of Gastroenterology recommends beginning the initial screening in blacks at age 45, because of an increased risk of colon cancer. Colonoscopy every 10 years is recommended after a normal colonoscopy. The US Preventive Services Task Force recommends against routine screening after age 75. The benefits of screening at that age are less than the risks of the screen, and the likelihood that a patient will die of another cause of death besides colon cancer.

A family history of colon cancer may result in recommendations to start screening at an earlier age. First-degree relatives with colorectal cancer or an advanced adenoma (eg, 10 mm or larger, villous elements, or high-grade dysplasia) before the age of 60 years or 2 second-degree relatives at any age with these risks should start screening at age 40 years or 10 years younger than the relative's age at diagnosis, whichever is earlier. Intervals for screening colonoscopy in this group should be every 5 years.

Besides finding early cancer, finding and treating colon polyps is an important benefit. There are 2 types of colon polyps: cancerous and noncancerous. Hyperplastic polyps are the most common type of noncancerous polyp. Finding a hyperplastic polyp in the rectum or the sigmoid does not indicate an increased risk of cancer; therefore, it is only necessary to repeat the colonoscopy in 10 years.

Adenomas are polyps with malignant potential; 75% of all colorectal cancers develop from adenomatous polyps. Different histologic types of adenomatous polyps differ in their degree of malignant potential. Tubular adenomas, accounting for 80% of adenomas, transform at a rate of 4.8%. The other adenomas, tubulovillous and villous, have greater malignant potential, transforming at a rate of 19.0% and 38.4%, respectively. Adenomas are graded on their degree of dysplasia, either low grade or high grade. Low-risk, small (<10 mm) tubular adenomas require a follow-up colonoscopy in 5 years. Repeat colonoscopy at 3 years is recommended for high-risk polyps, a single tubular or serrated polyp 10 mm or greater, a single polyp with villous or high-grade dysplasia, a single sessile serrated polyp with dysplasia, or a traditional serrated adenoma, or 3 to 10 tubular adenomas. Sessile polyps are more difficult to detect. They are flat, indiscrete, and often covered with adherent mucus. They are more dysplastic.

Although colonoscopy is the best screening test for colon cancer, it is not the only screening option. Regular FOBT is still in the US Preventive Services Task Force guideline recommendations. The rationale is that most cancers and large adenomas bleed intermittently. FOBT is better at detecting early cancers than adenomas. Annual testing is needed because testing every 2 years has found to be inadequate. Three samples should be collected at home. Stool from a digital rectal examination should not be used. Vitamin C should be avoided; it causes false negatives because it blocks peroxidase. False positives can occur with aspirin, NSAIDS, red meat, poultry, fish, and some raw vegetables. Annual testing has been shown in metaanalysis to decrease mortality by 16%.[55]

The fecal immunochemical test (FIT) checks for occult bleeding in a different way than the guaiac-based test. The FIT detects the hemoglobin protein, not peroxidase. It has no dietary or drug restrictions, unlike the FOBT. It requires 1 specimen rather than the 3 required by the FOBT. Compared with FOBT, FIT has a higher sensitivity for colorectal cancer (79% vs 20%–50%) and for advanced polyps (20%–50% vs 11%–20%).[56]

The use of double-contrast barium enemas seems to be decreasing, but is still included as a screening recommendation. The detection rates for adenomas larger than 10 mm is 48%. Fewer young radiologists are being trained in the procedure. No formal trial has been performed in the general population regarding outcomes.

Computed tomographic colonography requires bowel preparation and uses a very low dose of radiation. The test seems as good as colonoscopy in the detection of polyps.[57] It is unclear whether it can detect flat, serrated polyps, and it is uncertain how it reduces mortality compared with other screening methods. About 10% to 25% of those screened with computed tomographic colonography require referral for a colonoscopy, which then requires a second preparation, a second visit, and has an increased cost.

The most recently developed screening test is for stool DNA. It detects certain DNA mutations associated with cancer or polyps with these mutations. One manufacturer combines the DNA test with a test for blood. The sensitivity of the combined test to detect cancer and advance precancerous lesions is 20% better than the FIT alone, but is less specific.[58] Ten percent of the subjects that tested positive had entirely normal colonoscopies. This test should be done every 3 years. Any positive results requires colonoscopy. Because it is a relatively new test, some insurance companies may not cover it because the cost may be as high as $1000.

SUMMARY

The recommendation for screening, treatment, and prognosis varies between these 3 cancers, but a common theme prevails—a healthy lifestyle. Not smoking, maintaining an ideal body weight, moderation of alcohol use, regular exercise, and a diet rich in fruits and vegetables seem to reduce the risk of these cancers. One interesting exception is the acquisition of *H pylori*, which results in a lower risk of esophageal cancer. Solid guidelines are in place for colon cancer screening, but not for screening for esophageal or gastric cancers. Treatments for these cancers require multidisciplinary team work, and the family physician should be a key member of the team, active in the patient's entire disease process.

REFERENCES

1. National Cancer Institute, Surveillance, Epidemiology, and End Results Program. Cancer stat facts: esophageal cancer. Available at: http://seer.cancer.gov/statfacts/html/esoph.html. Accessed October 28, 2017.
2. American Cancer Society. Cancer facts and figures 2005. Atlanta (GA): American Cancer Society; 2005.
3. Rubenstein JH, Taylor JB. Meta-analysis: the association of oesophageal adenocarcinoma with symptoms of gastro-oesophageal reflux. Aliment Pharmacol Ther 2010;32:1222–7.

4. Zambon P, Talamini R, La Vecchia C, et al. Smoking, type of alcoholic beverage and squamous-cell oesophageal cancer in northern Italy. Int J Cancer 2000;86: 144–9.
5. Martin IG, Young S, Sue-Ling H, et al. Delays in the diagnosis of oesophagogastric cancer: a consecutive series. BMJ 1997;314:467–70.
6. Freeman HJ. Risk of gastrointestinal malignancies and mechanisms of cancer development with obesity and its treatment. Best Pract Res Clin Gastroenterol 2004;18:1167–75.
7. Blot WJ, Devesa SS, Kneller RW, et al. Rising incidence of adenocarcinoma of the esophagus and gastric cardia. JAMA 1991;265:1287–9.
8. Cook MB, Kamangar F, Whiteman DC, et al. Cigarette smoking and adenocarcinomas of the esophagus and esophagogastric junction: a pooled analysis from the international BEACON consortium. J Natl Cancer Inst 2010;102:1344–53.
9. Rustgi AK, El-Serag HB. Esophageal carcinoma. N Engl J Med 2014;371: 2499–509.
10. Xie FJ, Zhang YP, Zheng QQ, et al. Helicobacter pylori infection and esophageal cancer risk: an updated meta-analysis. World J Gastroenterol 2013;19:6098–107.
11. Rokkas T, Pistiolas D, Sechopoulos P, et al. Relationship between Helicobacter pylori infection and esophageal neoplasia: a meta-analysis. Clin Gastroenterol Hepatol 2007;5:1413–7.
12. Mayer RJ. Gastrointestinal tract cancer. In: Longo DL, Fauci AS, Kasper DL, et al, editors. Harrison's principles of internal medicine 1. 18th edition. Medical Publishing Division: New York: McGraw-Hill; 2012.
13. Hvid-Jensen F, Pedersen L, Drewes AM, et al. Incidence of adenocarcinoma among patients with Barrett's esophagus. N Engl J Med 2011;365:1375–83.
14. Shaheen NJ, Sharma P, Overholt BF, et al. Radiofrequency ablation in Barrett's esophagus with dysplasia. N Engl J Med 2009;360:2277–88.
15. Prevention: Dietary Factors, based on Chainani-Wu N. Diet and oral, pharyngeal, and esophageal cancer. Nutr Cancer 2002;44(2):104–26.
16. Coleman HG, Murray LJ, Hicks B, et al. Dietary fiber and the risk of precancerous lesions and cancer of the esophagus: a systematic review and meta-analysis. Nutr Rev 2013;71(7):474–82.
17. Kastelein F, Spaander MC, Steyerberg EW, et al. Proton pump inhibitors reduce the risk of neoplastic progression in patients with Barrett's esophagus. Clin Gastroenterol Hepatol 2013;11:382–8.
18. Singh S, Singh AG, Singh PP, et al. Statins are associated with reduced risk of esophageal cancer, particularly in patients with Barrett's esophagus: a systematic review and meta-analysis. Clin Gastroenterol Hepatol 2013;11:620–9.
19. Jemal A, Murray T, Samuels A, et al. Cancer statistics, 2003. CA Cancer J Clin 2003;53:5–26.
20. Tokui N, Yoshimura T, Fujino Y, et al. Dietary habits and stomach cancer risk in the JACC study. J Epidemiol 2005;15(Suppl II):S98–108.
21. Parsonnet J, Friedman G, Orentreich N, et al. Risk for gastric cancer in people with cag A positive or cag A negative Helicobacter pylori infection. Gut 1997; 40:297–301.
22. Fock KM, Talley N, Moayyedi P, et al. Asia-Pacific consensus guidelines on gastric cancer prevention. J Gastroenterol Hepatol 2008;23:351–65.
23. Helicobacter and Cancer Collaborative Group. Gastric cancer and Helicobacter pylori: a combined analysis of 12 case control studies nested within prospective cohorts. Gut 2001;49:347–53.

24. D'Elia L, Rossi G, Ippolito R, et al. Habitual salt intake and risk of gastric cancer: a meta-analysis of prospective studies. Clin Nutr 2012;31(4):489–98.
25. Lunet N, Lacerda-Vieira A, Barros H. Fruit and vegetables consumption and gastric cancer: a systematic review and meta-analysis of cohort studies. Nutr Cancer 2005;53:1–10.
26. Bertuccio P, Rosato V, Andreano A, et al. Dietary patterns and gastric cancer risk: a systematic review and meta-analysis. Ann Oncol 2013;24:1450–8.
27. Sasazuki S, Tamakoshi A, Matsuo K, et al. Green tea consumption and gastric cancer risk: an evaluation based on a systematic review of epidemiologic evidence among the Japanese population. Jpn J Clin Oncol 2012;42:335–46.
28. Ladeiras-Lopes R, Pereira AK, Nogueira A, et al. Smoking and gastric cancer: systematic review and meta-analysis of cohort studies. Cancer Causes Control 2008;19:689 701.
29. Yang P, Zhou Y, Chen B, et al. Overweight, obesity and gastric cancer risk: results from a meta-analysis of cohort studies. Eur J Cancer 2009;45:2867–73.
30. Shimazu T, Tsuji I, Inoue M, et al. Alcohol drinking and gastric cancer risk: an evaluation based on a systematic review of epidemiologic evidence among the Japanese population. Jpn J Clin Oncol 2008;38:8–25.
31. Weitzel JN. Genetic cancer risk assessment: putting it all together. Cancer 1999; 86:2483–92.
32. Allum WH, Blazeby JM, Griffin SM, et al. Guidelines for the management of oesophageal and gastric cancer. Gut 2011;60(11):1449–72.
33. National Comprehensive Cancer Network. Gastric cancer: version 3. 2015.
34. Memon MA, Subramanya MS, Khan S, et al. Meta-analysis of D1 versus D2 gastrectomy for gastric adenocarcinoma. Ann Surg 2011;253(5):900–11.
35. Sindelar WG, Kinsella TJ. Randomized trial of resection and intraoperative radiotherapy in locally advanced gastric cancer. Proc Ann Meet Am Soc Clin Oncol 1987;6:A357.
36. Allum WH, Hallissey MT, Ward LC, et al. A controlled, prospective, randomised trial of adjuvant chemotherapy or radiotherapy in resectable gastric cancer: interim report. British Stomach Cancer Group. Br J Cancer 1989;60(5):739–44.
37. American Cancer Society. Colorectal cancer facts and figures 2011-2013. Atlanta (GA): American Cancer Society; 2010.
38. Desch CE, Benson AB 3rd, Somerfield MR, et al. Colorectal cancer surveillance: 2005 update of an American Society of Clinical Oncology practice guideline. J Clin Oncol 2005;23(33):8512–9.
39. National Cancer Institute. SEER stat fact sheets: colon and rectum. 2011.
40. American Cancer Society. Cancer Facts. 2016.
41. Calle EE, Rodriguez C, Walker-Thurmond K, et al. Overweight, obesity, and mortality from cancer in a prospectively studied cohort of U.S. adults. N Engl J Med 2003;348:1625–38.
42. Slattery ML, Schumacher MC, Smith KR, et al. Physical activity, diet, and risk of colon cancer in Utah. Am J Epidemiol 1988;128:989–99.
43. Terry P, Giovannucci E, Michels KB, et al. Fruit, vegetables, dietary fiber, and risk of colorectal cancer. J Natl Cancer Inst 2001;93:525–33.
44. Terry MB, Neugut AI, Bostick RM, et al. Risk factors for advanced colorectal adenomas: a pooled analysis. Cancer Epidemiol Biomarkers Prev 2002;11:622–9.
45. Meyerhardt JA, Giovannucci EL, Holmes MD, et al. Physical activity and survival after colorectal cancer diagnosis. J Clin Oncol 2006;24:3527–34.

46. Giovannucci E. An updated review of the epidemiological evidence that cigarette smoking increases risk of colorectal cancer. Cancer Epidemiol Biomarkers Prev 2001;10(7):725–31.
47. Levin B, Ludwig KA, Steinbach G. Colorectal cancer screening. Clinical practice guidelines in oncology. J Natl Compr Canc Netw 2003;1(1):72–93.
48. Chlebowski RT, Wactawski-Wende J, Ritenbaugh C, et al. Estrogen plus progestin and colorectal cancer in postmenopausal women. N Engl J Med 2004;350: 991–1004.
49. Thun MJ, Namboodiri MM, Heath CW Jr. Aspirin use and reduced risk of fatal colon cancer. N Engl J Med 1991;325:1593–6.
50. Nishihara R, Wu K, Lochhead P, et al. Long-term colorectal-cancer incidence and mortality after lower endoscopy. N Engl J Med 2013;369:1095–105.
51. Shaukat A, Mongin SJ, Geisser MS, et al. Long-term mortality after screening for colorectal cancer. N Engl J Med 2013;369:1106–14.
52. Winawer SJ, Stewart ET, Zauber AG, et al. A comparison of colonoscopy and double-contrast barium enema for surveillance after polypectomy. National Polyp Study Work Group. N Engl J Med 2000;342:1766–72.
53. Klabunde CN, Vernon SW, Nadel MR, et al. Barriers to colorectal cancer screening: a comparison of reports from primary care physicians and average-risk adults. Med Care 2005;43:939–44.
54. Klabunde CN, Vernon SW, Nadel MR, et al. Center for Disease Control and Prevention (CDC) cancer screening-United States, 2010. MMWR Morb Mortal Wkly Rep 2012;61(3):41–5.
55. Hewitson P, Glasziou P, Irwig L, et al. Screening for colorectal cancer using the fecal occult blood test, hemoccult. Cochrane Database Syst Rev 2007;(1):CD001216.
56. Lee JK, Liles EG, Brent S, et al. Accuracy of fecal immunochemical tests for colorectal cancer: systematic review and meta-analysis. Ann Intern Med 2014;160(3): 171–81.
57. Johnson CD, Chen M-H, Toledano AY, et al. Accuracy of CT colonography for detection of large adenomas and cancers. N Engl J Med 2008;359(12):1207–17.
58. Thomas F, Ransohoff DF, Itzkowitz SH, et al. Multitarget stool DNA testing for colorectal-cancer screening. N Engl J Med 2014;370:1287–97.

Emerging Topics in Gastroenterology

Gretchen Irwin, MD, MBA, Laura Mayans, MD, MPH*, Rick Kellerman, MD

KEYWORDS

- Microbiome • Probiotics • Fecal transplant • Cyclic vomiting
- Eosinophilic esophagitis • Microscopic colitis

KEY POINTS

- Genetic variations, diet, stress, and medication use have all been demonstrated to affect the composition of the microbiota in the gastrointestinal tract. Aging may lead to changes in physiology that impact gastrointestinal bacteria, potentially resulting in somatic symptoms related to a disordered microbiome.
- Fecal microbiota transplantation (FMT) has been shown to significantly alter the composition of the recipient's gut microbiome.
- Cyclic Vomiting Syndrome episodes are often triggered by emotional stress or antecedent viral illnesses. CVS is a diagnosis of exclusion, as it lacks any identifying radiological or laboratory abnormalities.
- Eosinophilic esophagitis(EE) is an increasingly-recognized cause of dysphagia and food impaction as well as infant feeding problems.
- Microscopic colitis(MC) is microscopic inflammation of the colonic mucosa that can cause chronic, watery, non-bloody diarrhea, abdominal cramping, and pain. The cause of MC is unclear and it can only be diagnosed through biopsy of the colonic mucosa.

GASTROINTESTINAL MICROBIOME AND PROBIOTICS

Researchers estimate that more than 100 trillion bacteria representing more than 600 different phylotypes can be found within a healthy human gut.[1] Additionally, more than 30 different fungal species may also be found in humans, depending on gender and stage of life.[2] These bacteria and fungi make up a community of microorganisms that lives in symbiosis with humans, engaging in numerous diverse interactions that influence health. Though the gastrointestinal (GI) microbiome undoubtedly interacts with the human body, there is much that is unknown about the formation, maintenance, and impact that the microbiome has on health and disease.

The authors have nothing to disclose.
Department of Family and Community Medicine, University of Kansas School of Medicine-Wichita, 1010 North Kansas, Wichita, KS 67214, USA
* Corresponding author.
E-mail address: lmayans@kumc.edu

Prim Care Clin Office Pract 44 (2017) 733–742
http://dx.doi.org/10.1016/j.pop.2017.07.008
0095-4543/17/© 2017 Elsevier Inc. All rights reserved.

New evidence suggests that the microbiome begins forming during the fetal period either through translocation of bacteria from maternal circulation or colonization via bacterial ascension from the vagina.[3,4] The method of delivery and the first few days of life significantly modify the microbiome composition.[4] Early diet plays a key role in establishing a colony of good bacteria as human milk oligosaccharides found in breast milk stimulate the growth of key bacteria. Interestingly, randomized trials have demonstrated that the consumption of human milk oligosaccharide analogues, even by adults, can improve the microbiome by stimulating the growth of bifidobacteria.[5]

After establishment, the microbiome continues to evolve in composition and function throughout the first few years of life. During this period, enteric neurons, immunologic factors, and the microbiome itself interact through complex signaling pathways to establish a homeostatic environment in the GI tract.[6] By age 3 years, the microbiome takes on a composition with characteristics that remain generally consistent through much of adulthood.[4] However, many events can shift microbiome composition and function in ways that may ultimately affect health. For example, exposure to antibiotics in early childhood may lead to lifelong changes in the composition of the microbiome.[7,8] Also, as individuals choose a more restricted diet that eliminates specific animal or plant sources of food, the substrates available for bacteria within the GI system can change dramatically. Changing substrates may create new patterns of bacterial growth and changes in the diversity of the microbiome.[9] Genetic variations, diet, stress, and medication use have all been demonstrated to affect the composition of the microbiota in the GI tract.[8] Aging may lead to changes in physiology that affect GI bacteria, potentially resulting in somatic symptoms related to a disordered microbiome.[10,11]

Research is now focusing on the impact that an altered microbiome has on an individual's health and symptomatology. When the composition of the microbiome shifts, individuals may begin to experience specific pathologic symptoms. For example, in patients with irritable bowel syndrome, studies suggest that alterations in bacterial composition are associated with changes in epithelial barrier dysfunction, visceral hypersensitivity, and GI motility.[12,13]

However, GI symptoms, such as diarrhea, constipation, bloating, and abdominal pain, are no longer thought to be the only manifestations of a disordered microbiome. Dysbiosis, a condition wherein the healthy microbial structure of the GI tract is disturbed, has been postulated to be an inciting event or contributing factor to the development or worsening of metabolic disease, mental health, neurologic disease, and cancer, among other conditions.[12,14,15] For instance, children who are raised in homes with pets have alterations in their microbiome that may be a link to protection from developing allergic diseases and respiratory virus infections.[7] Furthermore, studies of individuals with atherosclerosis demonstrate that those with and without disease have significantly different bacterial species that predominate in their GI microbiome.[16] The combination of a specific microbiome composition with a diet that provides a specific digestive substrate may result in the synthesis of trimethylamine-N-oxide, which has been identified as a risk factor for major cardiovascular events.[16] Similarly, in 1 study, the gut microbiome composition was found to be more predictive of type 2 diabetes disease severity than the body mass index.[17] The microbiome is also different in obese and lean individuals.[18–20] These observations raise interesting questions for future research. Does the composition of the microbiome drive disease or does the disease state alter the milieu of the environment such that the microbiome composition changes? What is the clinical significance of knowing about an alteration? Can diagnostic strategies or treatment options be developed that allow clinicians to partner with the microbiome to improve disease outcomes?

Although metagenomics and emerging techniques targeted at taxonomic identification of gut bacterial composition have significantly increased knowledge of the GI microbiome, little is known about how to apply these observations to the diagnosis and treatment of clinical disease. Many associations are postulated, but few evidence-based recommendations can be made.

Nonetheless, probiotics have gained popularity as a potential source of restoring an ideal GI microbiome to improve symptoms, prevent illness, and treat disease. A meta-analysis of randomized controlled trials demonstrated that probiotic supplementation significantly improved low-density lipoprotein cholesterol levels, which may suggest a route for improving cardiac risk factors beyond current pharmacologic interventions.[21] Further, modulation of the microbiome through administration of probiotics has been demonstrated to help some individuals improve tolerance of medications such as metformin.[22] Several studies have suggested improved behavioral symptoms in children on the autism spectrum after administration of probiotics. The mechanism of action is postulated to be the result of alterations in neurochemical signals from bacteria in the gut that are transmitted through the microbiota-gut-brain axis.[23] Although these results are encouraging, they are very preliminary and are far from ready for widespread clinical implementation.

Probiotics have even been studied as a potential source of performance enhancement for athletes. Using mouse models, researchers have shown that the physical and emotional stress that occurs during exercise may alter the microbiome. This can result in a change of the neurotransmitters released by the gut that travel via enteric neurons to the brain. The changes in serotonin, dopamine, and other neurochemicals may lead to fatigue and mood disturbance, and manifest as underperformance. The question remains, however, if probiotic supplementation can positively affect the gut microbiome and result in the ideal neurotransmitter signals to optimize performance during training or competition.[24]

Although probiotics have been touted to improve the immune system, help prevent bowel disease, treat conditions ranging from lactose intolerance to hypertension, and even alleviate postmenopausal symptoms, much of the evidence of effectiveness is anecdotal.[25] Published clinical trials have been limited and show mixed results. For example, the use of probiotics to treat chronic GI diseases such as irritable bowel syndrome seems to make pathophysiologic sense, yet data are mixed when implemented clinically.[12,26] Similarly, a review of 2900 subjects in 30 trials demonstrated that probiotics significantly reduced nosocomial infections, including ventilator-associated pneumonia in critically ill subjects. However, no reduction was noted in mortality or length of stay, making clinical application of these findings difficult.[27]

Moreover, as a supplement, probiotics lack standard formulations and dosages, which further impairs clinical use even when research has demonstrated effectiveness. For example, probiotics have been shown to be effective for the prevention and treatment of antibiotic-associated diarrhea, yet the lack of standardization of supplements makes clinical implementation of this knowledge difficult.[28] Research suggests that a diverse diet, rich in fiber, provides an optimized environment to stimulate growth and activity of the ideal microbiome. This may be as effective as supplementation with probiotics, which may or may not contain the ideal bacteria needed by a given individual.[8,10]

FECAL MICROBIOTA TRANSPLANTATION

Collectively, these organisms that make up the gut microbiome have more than 100 times more genes than their human host. Emerging research suggests these microorganisms and their collective genome may play an important role in metabolic health and disease.[29] The gut microbiome can be altered in multiple ways. In addition to the ingestion of probiotics and prebiotics, the transplantation of fecal matter can also alter the gut microbiome. Attempts to change an individual's gut microbiome go back as far as the fourth century when the first fecal transplant was recorded for the treatment of severe diarrhea.[29]

Fecal microbiota transplantation (FMT) has been shown to significantly alter the composition of the recipient's gut microbiome. Randomized controlled trials have demonstrated the success of FMT in the treatment of recurrent or refractory *Clostridium difficile* infection, which is the only application of FMT approved by the US Food and Drug Administration (FDA).[29–31] Research continues into the best delivery method for FMT in the treatment of *C difficile* infections, as well as the use of FMT in several other conditions, including vancomycin-resistant *Enterococcus* (VRE) infection and the treatment of obesity and metabolic syndrome.[29–33]

FMT in *C difficile* infection has been highly effective (83%–100%) and rarely associated with major adverse events.[31] However, its use is limited by practical barriers and stigma. Currently, donor stool is collected, processed, and suspended in sterile saline.[30] It is then delivered via nasogastric tube, upper endoscopy, or in a retrograde fashion via colonoscopy, all with similar success rates.[31] These methods all expose patients to risk, as well as discomfort. Delivery of FMT using oral capsules of frozen fecal material is being investigated at Massachusetts General Hospital.[30] Subjects are given 15 capsules on 2 consecutive days (30 capsules total). To date, 202 subjects have been treated and 180 have had documented follow-up. *C difficile* infections resolved in 82% of subjects after a single treatment and 91% with 2 treatments. These rates are in line with endoscopic and colonoscopic administration of FMT. Though promising, more study is needed to document long-term safety.

FMT is also being studied for VRE, as well as obesity and metabolic syndrome. Data are still primarily from animal studies. Studies of FMT in VRE-colonized mice have shown some promise, but case studies in human subjects have not been as successful.[32,33] Studies conducted in rodents have suggested that FMT has the ability to alter the metabolic phenotype of the recipient.[29] Mice receiving an FMT from an obese rat demonstrated increased adiposity compared with those receiving it from a lean rat. One published study examined the efficacy of FMT in metabolic syndrome in humans.[29] The study involved 18 subjects and, although there was no significant body mass index difference between groups at 6 weeks, there was a statistically significant increase in insulin sensitivity. Clinicaltrials.gov lists several other ongoing trials involving FMT. Studies in the United States, Italy, China, and Canada are examining the effect of FMT on body weight reduction, glucose homeostasis, type 2 diabetes, metabolic syndrome, and nonalcoholic fatty liver disease.

Important research questions about FMT exist. Who is the ideal donor, who is the ideal recipient, how long do gut microbiome alterations persist, and does FMT have applications beyond treatment of GI infections? These questions and more are subject to hypothesis generation and continuing research.

CYCLIC VOMITING SYNDROME

Cyclic vomiting syndrome (CVS), first described in 1882, is a poorly understood functional GI disorder characterized by recurrent bouts of nausea and severe vomiting, with a return to baseline health between episodes. It was long thought to occur primarily in children but is now known to occur in adults as well. The median age of onset is between 4 and 7 years, and the incidence is estimated to be 3.2 per 100,000 children per year.[34]

The underlying causes of CVS are unknown but believed to be similar to other triggered, episodic disorders such as migraine, epilepsy, and panic disorders.[35] Some cases are believed to be related to mitochondrial dysfunction and many investigators believe CVS is a form of abdominal migraine because cases are frequently associated with migraine headaches.[34] Approximately 30% of children with CVS will continue to experience episodes into adulthood.[34] Children with CVS will typically have 8 to 12 attacks per year characterized by severe vomiting, often with at least 4 episodes per hour.[34] An attack will usually last 20 to 48 hours in children, longer in adults. Vomiting often begins in the early morning hours and more than 70% of episodes are associated with abdominal pain. Episodes are often triggered by emotional stress or antecedent viral illnesses. CVS is a diagnosis of exclusion because it lacks any identifying radiological or laboratory abnormalities.

Treatment of CVS consists of 2 parts: aborting acute attacks and prophylaxis of future attacks. Acute treatment is aimed at controlling nausea and vomiting, and addressing fluid status and electrolyte imbalances. In many ways, acute treatment is similar to that for acute migraine. Patients should lie down in a quiet, dark room. 5-Hydroxytryptamine type 3 (5-HT$_3$) receptor antagonists such as ondansetron are the mainstay of treatment of nausea and vomiting.[34] Triptans can also be tried, especially in attacks associated with migraine headaches. Isotonic saline boluses are used to restore hydration, followed by dextrose-containing solution until the patient can tolerate oral intake. Patients rarely require hospitalization unless they have lost greater than 5% fluid volume, have been anuric for 12 hours or more, have severe metabolic or electrolyte disturbances, or are unable to control emesis.[34] Amitriptyline and beta-blockers have been the mainstays of prophylactic treatment, though recent studies have shown promising, and improved, results with topiramate.[34,36] Psychological factors also play a role in CVS, both as a trigger and as a cause of worsened disability from the disorder.[37] Therefore, a biopsychosocial approach that also uses psychotherapy can be useful in CVS.

There is a high incidence of clinical anxiety in children with CVS. Children with diagnosed or suspected CVS should be screened for anxiety and, if present, treated appropriately.[38] Treatment of coexisting anxiety can help improve the child's coping ability, if not the disorder itself. In adults, an increasingly identified cause of CVS is overuse of cannabis.[34] Low dose use of cannabis can have antiemetic effects, but chronic, frequent use can have the opposite effect. Cannabinoid hyperemesis syndrome is characterized by cyclic and recurrent vomiting, abdominal pain, and the unusual feature of taking frequent, hot showers that seem to ameliorate symptoms. Cessation of cannabis use usually aborts the attack.

EOSINOPHILIC ESOPHAGITIS

Eosinophilic esophagitis, once considered to be a rare condition, is increasingly diagnosed.[39] It is unclear if eosinophilic esophagitis is increasing in prevalence or if it was previously under-recognized. The diagnosis is made by observing 15 eosinophils per high-power field on a biopsy specimen of the esophagus. The male to female ratio is 3:1 and it is most common in white men.[40]

Eosinophilic esophagitis can be asymptomatic; it can also cause dysphagia and food impaction. It is reported that up to 54% of patients undergoing endoscopy for a history of food impaction in the esophagus are discovered to have eosinophilic esophagitis.[41] In the absence of a clear reason for dysphagia or esophageal food impaction, a biopsy of the esophagus should be strongly considered to aid in making a diagnosis.

The cause of eosinophilic esophagitis is thought to be immune-mediated and the antigens responsible for the immune response seem to be food-based. There are several interesting theories on why eosinophilic esophagitis seems to be increasing in prevalence. Many of these theories revolve around the hygiene hypothesis. The hygiene hypothesis postulates that a lack of early childhood exposure to various microorganisms and allergens suppress the natural development of the immune system. Lack of exposure to these agents may lead to defects in immune tolerance. Antibiotic exposure during infancy, food allergy, and a lack of breastfeeding are associated with eosinophilic esophagitis.[42] There may be a positive family history of eosinophilic esophagitis or a family history of atopic disorders such as asthma, eczema, or anaphylaxis.[43]

On visual inspection of the esophageal mucosa of patients with eosinophilic esophagitis, the mucosa may demonstrate small white specks that represent eosinophilic exudates. There may also be evidence of strictures, linear furrows in the mucosa, and mucosal edema.[43] When the endoscopist performs a mucosal biopsy, she or he may notice some resistance when taking the biopsy specimen; this has come to be known as the tug sign.[44] Linear tears in the esophagus may occur with minimal trauma during passage of the endoscope. A barium swallow complements the evaluation of eosinophilic esophagitis because some strictures in this condition may be lengthy and tapered and, therefore, may not be evident on direct observation with the endoscope.[43]

The most effective treatment of eosinophilic esophagitis is an elemental diet consisting of amino acids and the elimination of food antigens.[45,46] This dietary regimen almost completely eliminates the symptoms of eosinophilic esophagitis and histologic abnormalities. Unfortunately, many patients cannot abide by a strict elemental diet. Using skin-prick allergy testing, patch testing, and serum IgE testing to identify specific allergens and guide the focused elimination of foods has had disappointing results.[45] Another option is to empirically avoid the 6 most common allergenic foods: wheat, milk, soy, nuts, eggs, and seafood, the so-called 6-food elimination diet.[43,46] In general, acid suppression with proton pump inhibitors and histamine blockers does not help, though they are frequently prescribed.[43] Though not approved by the FDA, a fluticasone metered-dose inhaler and a viscous preparation of liquid budesonide have been tried in some research studies with some evidence of symptom and histologic improvement.[40,43,45,46] Esophageal dilation may be required in some patients with luminal narrowing due to eosinophilic esophagitis.[43,45,46] Antireflux surgical procedures have not been shown to help.[43]

Current evidence does not indicate that eosinophilic esophagitis is a premalignant syndrome and it does not seem to shorten lifespan. However, it does seem to be a chronic disease and complications such as esophageal strictures may develop.[43]

Eosinophilic esophagitis can also cause infant feeding problems. Symptoms include a wide variety of nonspecific feeding problems, such as vomiting and failure to thrive, in infants. Children may suffer from nausea, vomiting, and abdominal pain. Teenagers and young adults can suffer nausea, vomiting, and abdominal pain, as well as food impaction, dysphagia, and reflux symptoms.[47] It has been proposed that children, adolescents, and young adults with eosinophilic esophagitis learn to compensate for their symptoms by eating slowly, chewing carefully, cutting food into small pieces, and drinking lots of fluids when they eat to lubricate and dilute foods. They may avoid some foods, such as meat and bread, and may avoid eating in public or taking pills. It is postulated that some patients have years and years of silent or subclinical disease by almost unconsciously controlling their symptoms with these techniques.[43]

MICROSCOPIC COLITIS

As the name implies, microscopic colitis is inflammation of the colon that is only apparent on histologic evaluation of tissue.[48,49] Symptoms most commonly associated with microscopic colitis are chronic, watery, nonbloody diarrhea and abdominal cramping and pain. Patients may have 5 to 10 watery stools per day. Symptoms can last for days to months or years, or can be intermittent. Bloating, nausea, and rectal urgency may also be present. Rarely, fecal incontinence and weight loss may occur.[49]

A relationship between microscopic colitis and irritable bowel syndrome has been postulated. The relationship of microscopic colitis to inflammatory bowel disease is unclear. There are 2 subtypes of microscopic colitis. The first subtype, lymphocytic colitis, demonstrates an increase in lymphocytes in the mucosa, but the mucosal lining is of normal thickness. In the second subtype, collagenous colitis, lymphocytic infiltration is accompanied by collagen deposition in the mucosa and the mucosal lining may be thicker than usual. Whether these 2 subtypes are distinct entities or phases of the same condition is unclear. An individual may have findings of lymphocytic colitis and collagenous colitis in different parts of the colon.[48,49]

There are no blood tests, stool tests, imaging studies, or pathognomonic physical examination findings diagnostic of microscopic colitis. It can only be diagnosed with a biopsy of the colonic mucosa. A variety of laboratory tests, including sedimentation rate, peripheral blood eosinophil count, and serum complement levels, may be abnormal in a particular patient, but there are no definitive diagnostic markers.[48] An increased number of leukocytes may be identified in stool specimens. A few patients may have edema and mucosal erythema or paleness on visual inspection.[50]

The cause of microscopic colitis is unknown. It may be the result of an autoimmune reaction or an abnormal immune response to bacteria, medication, toxins, or noxious agents such as bile acid. The role of genetics is unclear.[48] A leading theory is that microscopic colitis develops after a bout of bacterial or viral gastroenteritis.[48] Autoimmune disorders associated with microscopic colitis include diabetes mellitus, celiac disease, thyroid disease, and rheumatoid arthritis.[48,49] The ingestion of many commonly used medications, such as nonsteroidal anti-inflammatory agents, proton pump inhibitors, histamine (H)-2 blockers, statins, and selective serotonin reuptake inhibitors, have been associated with microscopic colitis, but the causal link is unproven.[49,51] Risk factors for the development of microscopic colitis are age older than 50 years, female gender, underlying autoimmune disease, cigarette smoking, and use of medications associated with the disease. Children are rarely affected.[51,52]

Treatment includes discontinuation of tobacco smoking and, if possible, medications that might be related. Avoidance of symptom-inducing foods and beverages and use of symptom control medications, such as anti-diarrheal agents, may be used. Control of any underlying autoimmune disorders may be helpful. In some patients, cholestyramine resin can be helpful.[53–55] Budesonide rapidly induces symptom improvement but the relapse rate after discontinuation is high.[49,55,56] Evidence that the use of immune system modulators, anti-tumor necrosis factor (TNF) therapies, or biological agents is lacking and use of these agents should be driven by clinical judgment and balanced against the potential for treatment complications.[55] It does not seem that microscopic colitis increases the risk of colon cancer.[51]

REFERENCES

1. Schultz C, Schutte K, Koch N, et al. The active bacterial assemblages of the upper GI tract in individuals with and without *Helicobacter* infection. Gut 2016. [Epub ahead of print].

2. Strati F, DiPaola M, Stefanini I, et al. Age and gender affect the composition of fungal population of the human gastrointestinal tract. Front Microbiol 2016;7:1227.
3. Stinson LF, Payne MS, Keelan JA. Planting the seed: origins, composition and postnatal health significant of the fetal gastrointestinal microbiota. Crit Rev Microbiol 2017;43(3):352–69.
4. Brunst KJ, Wright RO, Digioia K, et al. Racial/ethnic and sociodemographic factors associated with micronutrient intakes and inadequacies among pregnant women in an urban US population. Public Health Nutr 2013;13:1–11.
5. Elison E, Vigsnaes LK, Rindom Krogsgaard L, et al. Oral supplementation of healthy adults with 2'-O-fucosyllactose and lacto-N-neotetraose is well tolerated and shifts the intestinal microbiota. Br J Nutr 2016;116(8):1356–68.
6. Obata Y, Pachnis V. The effect of microbiota and the immune system on the development and organization of the enteric nervous system. Gastroenterology 2016;151(5):836–44.
7. Slattery J, MacFabe D, Frye R. The significance of the enteric microbiome on the development of childhood disease: a review of prebiotic and probiotic therapies in disorders of childhood. Clin Med Insights Pediatr 2016;10:91–107.
8. Ericsson AC, Franklin CL. Manipulating the gut microbiota: methods and challenges. ILAR J 2015;56(2):205–17.
9. Heiman ML, Greenway FL. A healthy gastrointestinal microbiome is dependent on dietary diversity. Mol Metab 2016;5(5):317–20.
10. Claesson MJ, Jeffery IB, Conde S, et al. Gut microbiota composition correlates with diet and health in the elderly. Nature 2012;488(7410):178–84.
11. Kumar M, Babaei P, Ji B, et al. Human gut microbiota and healthy aging: Recent developments and future prospective. Nutr Healthy Aging 2016;4(1):3–16.
12. Nagao-Kitamoto H, Kitamoto S, Kuffa P, et al. Pathogenic role of the gut microbiota in gastrointestinal diseases. Intest Res 2016;14(2):127–38.
13. Bhattarai Y, Muniz Pedrogo DA, Kashyap PC. Irritable bowel syndrome: a gut microbiota-related disorder? Am J Physiol Gastrointest Liver Physiol 2017;312(1):G52–62.
14. Zhu Z, Xiong S, Liu D. The gastrointestinal tract: an initial organ of metabolic hypertension? Cell Physiol Biochem 2016;38(5):1681–94.
15. Mangiola F, Ianiro G, Franceschi F, et al. Gut microbiota in autism and mood disorders. World J Gastroenterol 2016;22(1):361–8.
16. Brown JM, Hazen SL. Metaorganismal nutrient metabolism as a basis of cardiovascular disease. Curr Opin Lipidol 2014;25(1):48–53.
17. Karlsson FH, Tremaroli V, Nookaew I, et al. Gut metagenome in European women with normal, impaired and diabetic glucose control. Nature 2013;498(7452):99–103.
18. Clarke SF, Murphy EF, Nilaweera K, et al. The gut microbiota and its relationship to diet and obesity: new insights. Gut Microbes 2012;3(3):186–202.
19. Vrieze A, Van Nood E, Holleman F, et al. Transfer of intestinal microbiota from lean donors increases insulin sensitivity in individuals with metabolic syndrome. Gastroenterology 2012;143(4):913–6.
20. Furet JP, Kong LC, Tap J, et al. Differential adaptation of human gut microbiota to bariatric surgery-induced weight loss: links with metabolic and low-grade inflammation markers. Diabetes 2010;59(12):3049–57.
21. Sharma S, Kurpad AV, Puri S. Potential of probiotics in hypercholesterolemia: a meta-analysis. Indian J Public Health 2016;60(4):280–6.

22. Bonnet F, Scheen A. Understanding and overcoming metformin gastrointestinal intolerance. Diabetes Obes Metab 2017;19(4):473–81.
23. Umbello G, Esposito S. Microbiota and neurologic diseases: potential effects of probiotics. J Transl Med 2016;14(1):298.
24. Clark A, Mach N. Exercise-induced stress behavior, gut-microbiota-brain axis and diet: a systematic review for athletes. J Int Soc Sports Nutr 2016;13:43.
25. Shi LH, Balakrishnan K, Thiagarajah K, et al. Beneficial properties of probiotics. Trop Life Sci Res 2016;27(2):73–90.
26. Imperatore N, Tortora R, Morisco F, et al. Review: gut microbiota and functional diseases of the gastrointestinal tract. Minerva Gastroenterol Dietol 2016. [Epub ahead of print].
27. Manzanares W, Lemieux M, Langlois P, et al. Probiotic and symbiotic therapy in critical illness: a systematic review and meta-analysis. Crit Care 2016;20:262.
28. Rodgers B, Kirley K, Mounsey A. Prescribing an antibiotic? Pair it with probiotics. J Fam Pract 2013;62(3):148–50.
29. Marotz CA, Azrrinpar A. Treating obesity and metabolic syndrome with fecal microbiota transplantation. Yale J Biol Med 2016;89:383–8.
30. Youngster I, Mahabamunuge J, Systrom HK, et al. Oral, frozen fecal microbiota transplant (FMT) capsules for Recurrent *Clostridium difficile* infection. BMC Med 2016;14:134–7.
31. Chapman BC, Moore HB, Overbey DM, et al. Fecal microbiota transplant in patients with *Clostridium difficile* infection: a systematic review. J Trauma Acute Care Surg 2016;81(4):756–64.
32. Sohn KM, Cheon S, Kim Y. Can fecal microbiota transplantation (FMT) eradicate fecal colonization with vancomycin-resistant enterococci (VRE)? Infect Control Hosp Epidemiol 2016;37(12):1519–21.
33. Ubeda C, Bucci V, Caballero S, et al. Intestinal microbiota containing *Barnesiella* species cures vancomycin-resistant *Enterococcus faecium* colonization. Infect Immun 2013;81:965–73.
34. Nagarwala J, Dev S, Markin A. The vomiting patient: small bowel obstruction, cyclic vomiting, and gastroparesis. Emerg Med Clin North Am 2016;34:271–91.
35. Levinthal DJ. The cyclic vomiting syndrome threshold: a framework for understanding pathogenesis and predicting successful treatment. Clin Transl Gastroenterol 2016;7:e198–205.
36. Sezer OB, Sezer T. A new approach to the prophylaxis of cyclic vomiting: topiramate. J Neurogastroenterol Motil 2016;22(4):656–60.
37. Reed-Knight B, Claar RL, Schurman JV, et al. Implementing psychological therapies for functional GI disorders in children and adults. Expert Rev Gastroenterol Hepatol 2016;10(9):981–4.
38. Tarbell SE, Millar A, Laudenslager M, et al. Anxiety and physiological responses to the trier social stress test for children and adolescents with cyclic vomiting syndrome. Auton Neurosci 2016. http://dx.doi.org/10.1016/j.autneu.2016.08.010.
39. Attwood S, Sabri S. Historical aspects of eosinophilic esophagitis: from case reports to clinical trials. Dig Dis 2014;32:34–9.
40. Dellon ES. Diagnosis and management of eosinophilic esophagitis. Clin Gastroenterol Hepatol 2012;10:1066–78.
41. Desai TK, Stecevic V, Chang CH, et al. Association of eosinophilic inflammation with esophageal food impaction in adults. Gastroentest Endosc 2005;61:795–801.
42. Jensen ET, Kappelman MD, Kim HP, et al. Early life exposures as risk factors for pediatric eosinophilic esophagitis. J Pediatr Gastroenterol Nutr 2013;57:67–71.

43. Furuta GT, Katzka DA. Eosinophilic esophagitis. N Engl J Med 2015;373(17): 1640–8.
44. Moawad FJ, Robinson CL, Veerappan GR, et al. The tug sign: an endoscopic feature of eosinophilic esophagitis (letter). Am J Gastroenterol 2013;252:1938–9.
45. Dellon ES, Gonsalves N, Hirano I, et al, American College of Gastroenterology. ACG clinical guidelines: evidence based approach to the diagnosis and management of esophageal eosinophilia and eosinophilic esophagitis (EoE). Am J Gastroenterol 2013;108:679–92.
46. Gonzalez-Cervera J, Lucendo AJ. Eosinophilic esophagitis: an evidence-based approach to therapy. J Investig Allergol Clin Immunol 2016;26(1):8–18.
47. Liacouras CA, Furuta GT, Hirano I, et al. Eosinophilic esophagitis: updated consensus recommendations for children and adults. J Allergy Clin Immunol 2011;128(1):3–20.e6.
48. Bohr J, Wickbom A, Hegedus A, et al. Diagnosis and management of microscopic colitis: current perspectives. Clin Exp Gastroenterol 2014;7:273–84.
49. Munch A, Aust D, Bohr J, et al, European Microscopic Colitis Group (EMCG). Microscopic colitis: current status, present and future challenges: statements of the European microscopic colitis group. J Crohns Colitis 2012;(6):932–45.
50. Park YS, Kim TK. Is microscopic colitis really microscopic? Gut Liver 2015;9(2): 137–8.
51. Storr MA. Microscopic colitis: epidemiology, pathophysiology, diagnosis and current management—an update 2013. ISRN Gastroenterol 2013;2013:352718.
52. Pisani LF, Tontini GE, Vecchi M, et al. Microscopic colitis: what do we know about pathogenesis? Inflamm Bowel Dis 2016;22(2):450–8.
53. Ohlsson B. New insights and challenges in microscopic colitis. Therap Adv Gastroenterol 2015;8(1):37–47.
54. Gentile NM, Abdalla AA, Khanna S, et al. Outcomes of patients with microscopic colitis treated with corticosteroids: a population-based study. Am J Gastroenterol 2013;108(2):256–9.
55. Park T, Cave D, Marshall C. Microscopic colitis: a review of etiology, treatment and refractory disease. World J Gastroenterol 2015;21(29):8804–10.
56. Chande N, MacDonald JK, McDonald JW. Interventions for treating microscopic colitis: a cochrane inflammatory bowel disease and functional bowel disorders review group systematic review of randomized trials. Am J Gastroenterol 2009; 104(1):235–41.

1. Publication Title	2. Publication Number	3. Filing Date
PRIMARY CARE: CLINICS IN OFFICE PRACTICE	044 – 690	9/18/2017

4. Issue Frequency	5. Number of Issues Published Annually	6. Annual Subscription Price
MAR, JUN, SEP, DEC	4	$232.00

7. Complete Mailing Address of Known Office of Publication (Not printer) (Street, city, county, state, and ZIP+4®)

ELSEVIER INC.
230 Park Avenue, Suite 800
New York, NY 10169

Contact Person
STEPHEN R. BUSHING

Telephone (Include area code)
215-239-3688

8. Complete Mailing Address of Headquarters or General Business Office of Publisher (Not printer)

ELSEVIER INC.
230 Park Avenue, Suite 800
New York, NY 10169

9. Full Names and Complete Mailing Addresses of Publisher, Editor, and Managing Editor (Do not leave blank)

Publisher (Name and complete mailing address)

ADRIANNE BRIGIDO ELSEVIER INC.
1600 JOHN F KENNEDY BLVD. SUITE 1800
PHILADELPHIA, PA 19103-2899

Editor (Name and complete mailing address)

JESSICA MCCOOL, ELSEVIER INC.
1600 JOHN F KENNEDY BLVD. SUITE 1800
PHILADELPHIA, PA 19103-2899

Managing Editor (Name and complete mailing address)

PATRICK MANLEY, ELSEVIER INC.
1600 JOHN F KENNEDY BLVD. SUITE 1800
PHILADELPHIA, PA 19103-2899

10. Owner (Do not leave blank. If the publication is owned by a corporation, give the name and address of the corporation immediately followed by the names and addresses of all stockholders owning or holding 1 percent or more of the total amount of stock. If not owned by a corporation, give the names and addresses of the individual owners. If owned by a partnership or other unincorporated firm, give its name and address as well as those of each individual owner. If the publication is published by a nonprofit organization, give its name and address.)

Full Name	Complete Mailing Address
WHOLLY OWNED SUBSIDIARY OF REED/ELSEVIER, US HOLDINGS	1600 JOHN F KENNEDY BLVD. SUITE 1800 PHILADELPHIA, PA 19103-2899

11. Known Bondholders, Mortgagees, and Other Security Holders Owning or Holding 1 Percent or More of Total Amount of Bonds, Mortgages, or Other Securities. If none, check box ▶ ☐ None

Full Name	Complete Mailing Address
N/A	

12. Tax Status (For completion by nonprofit organizations authorized to mail at nonprofit rates) (Check one)
The purpose, function, and nonprofit status of this organization and the exempt status for federal income tax purposes:
☒ Has Not Changed During Preceding 12 Months
☐ Has Changed During Preceding 12 Months (Publisher must submit explanation of change with this statement)

13. Publication Title	14. Issue Date for Circulation Data Below
PRIMARY CARE: CLINICS IN OFFICE PRACTICE	JUNE 2017

15. Extent and Nature of Circulation			Average No. Copies Each Issue During Preceding 12 Months	No. Copies of Single Issue Published Nearest to Filing Date
a. Total Number of Copies (Net press run)			142	93
b. Paid Circulation (By Mail and Outside the Mail)	(1)	Mailed Outside-County Paid Subscriptions Stated on PS Form 3541 (Include paid distribution above nominal rate, advertiser's proof copies, and exchange copies)	67	60
	(2)	Mailed In-County Paid Subscriptions Stated on PS Form 3541 (Include paid distribution above nominal rate, advertiser's proof copies, and exchange copies)	0	0
	(3)	Paid Distribution Outside the Mails Including Sales Through Dealers and Carriers, Street Vendors, Counter Sales, and Other Paid Distribution Outside USPS®	17	16
	(4)	Paid Distribution by Other Classes of Mail Through the USPS (e.g. First-Class Mail®)	0	0
c. Total Paid Distribution (Sum of 15b (1), (2), (3), and (4))			84	76
d. Free or Nominal Rate Distribution (By Mail and Outside the Mail)	(1)	Free or Nominal Rate Outside-County Copies included on PS Form 3541	29	17
	(2)	Free or Nominal Rate In-County Copies Included on PS Form 3541	0	0
	(3)	Free or Nominal Rate Copies Mailed at Other Classes Through the USPS (e.g. First-Class Mail)	0	0
	(4)	Free or Nominal Rate Distribution Outside the Mail (Carriers or other means)	0	0
e. Total Free or Nominal Rate Distribution (Sum of 15d (1), (2), (3) and (4))			29	17
f. Total Distribution (Sum of 15c and 15e)			113	93
g. Copies not Distributed (See Instructions to Publishers #4 (page #3))			29	0
h. Total (Sum of 15f and g)			142	93
i. Percent Paid (15c divided by 15f times 100)			74.34%	81.72%

* If you are claiming electronic copies, go to line 16 on page 3. If you are not claiming electronic copies, skip to line 17 on page 3.

16. Electronic Copy Circulation	Average No. Copies Each Issue During Preceding 12 Months	No. Copies of Single Issue Published Nearest to Filing Date
a. Paid Electronic Copies	▶ 0	0
b. Total Paid Print Copies (Line 15c) + Paid Electronic Copies (Line 16a)	▶ 84	76
c. Total Print Distribution (Line 15f) + Paid Electronic Copies (Line 16a)	▶ 113	93
d. Percent Paid (Both Print & Electronic Copies) (16b divided by 16c × 100)	▶ 74.34%	81.72%

☒ I certify that 50% of all my distributed copies (electronic and print) are paid above a nominal price.

17. Publication of Statement of Ownership

☒ If the publication is a general publication, publication of this statement is required. Will be printed ☐ Publication not required.
in the DECEMBER 2017 issue of this publication.

18. Signature and Title of Editor, Publisher, Business Manager, or Owner

STEPHEN R. BUSHING - INVENTORY DISTRIBUTION CONTROL MANAGER

Stephen R. Bushing (signature) Date 9/18/2017

I certify that all information furnished on this form is true and complete. I understand that anyone who furnishes false or misleading information on this form or who omits material or information requested on the form may be subject to criminal sanctions (including fines and imprisonment) and/or civil sanctions (including civil penalties).

Moving?

Make sure your subscription moves with you!

To notify us of your new address, find your **Clinics Account Number** (located on your mailing label above your name), and contact customer service at:

Email: **journalscustomerservice-usa@elsevier.com**

800-654-2452 (subscribers in the U.S. & Canada)
314-447-8871 (subscribers outside of the U.S. & Canada)

Fax number: **314-447-8029**

Elsevier Health Sciences Division
Subscription Customer Service
3251 Riverport Lane
Maryland Heights, MO 63043

*To ensure uninterrupted delivery of your subscription, please notify us at least 4 weeks in advance of move.